HEALTH CARE MARKETING

Issues and Trends

Edited by
Philip D. Cooper, Ph.D.

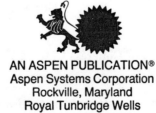

AN ASPEN PUBLICATION®
Aspen Systems Corporation
Rockville, Maryland
Royal Tunbridge Wells
1979

362.1
H44

Library of Congress Cataloging in Publication Data

Main entry under title:
Health care marketing.

Includes bibliographical references and index.

1. Medical care—Marketing—Addresses, essays,
lectures.   I. Cooper, Philip D., 1942-
[DNLM: WX157.3 H434]
RA410.5.H4   658.8'09'3621   79-18447
ISBN 0-89443-162-5

Library of Congress Catalog Card Number: 79-18447
ISBN: 0-89443-162-5

Printed in the United States of America

5

CONTENTS

CONTRIBUTORS

ERIC N. BERKOWITZ
Assistant Professor
Graduate School of Business
University of Minnesota
Minneapolis, Minnesota

SHIRLEY BONNEM
Associate Vice President and
Director Public Relations
The Children's Hospital of
Philadelphia
Philadelphia, Pennsylvania

RAY E. BROWN (deceased)
Executive Vice President
McGraw Medical Center
Northwestern University
Chicago, Illinos

F. TONY BUSHMAN
Assistant Professor
Department of Marketing
Drexel University
Philadelphia, Pennsylvania

ROBERT BYRNE
Director, Planning &
Development
Providence Memorial Hospital
El Paso, Texas

JAMES E. CASSIDY
Assistant Administrator
Metropolitan Hospital Center
New York, New York

PAUL CHIAMPA
School of Business
Administration
University of Virginia
Charlottesville, Virginia

ROBERTA CLARKE
Assistant Professor
Health Care Management
Program
Boston University
Boston, Massachusetts

ANTHONY CONSTANTINE
Assistant Commissioner of
Hospitals
New York City
New York, New York

LAMAR EKBLADH
Staff Physician
Department of Obstetrics &
Gynecology
North Carolina Memorial
Hospital
Chapel Hill, North Carolina

WILLIAM A. FLEXNER
Lecturer
Center for Health Services
Research
University of Minnesota
Minneapolis, Minnesota

TIM GARTON
Research Projects Director
Illinois Hospital Association
Oak Brook, Illinois

MARSHALL P. GAVIN
President
Primecare
Marina del Rey, California

C. T. HARDY
Assistant Clinic Manager
Watson Clinic
Lakeland, Florida

RICHARD C. IRELAND
Vice President of Marketing &
Development
Saint Joseph Hospital
Denver, Colorado

DAVID D. KARR
Vice President, Operations
Universal Health Services, Inc.
King of Prussia, Pennsylvania

WILLIAM J. KEHOE
Associate Professor
McIntire School of Commerce
University of Virginia
Charlottesville, Virginia

JAMES E. LITTLEFIELD
Professor
College of Business
Administration
University of North Carolina
Chapel Hill, North Carolina

CHRISTOPHER H. LOVELOCK
Associate Professor
Harvard Business School
Boston, Massachusetts

KEMSEY J. MACKEY
Associate Director, Mental
Health Services
St. Clare's Hospital
Denville, New Jersey

ROBIN E. MACSTRAVIC
Director
Program in Health Services
Administration
University of Washington
Seattle, Washington

CHRISTY MARSHALL
Associate Editor
Crain Communications
Chicago, Illinois

RICHARD B. MAXWELL, III
Vice President
Lakeview Medical Center
Danville, Illinois

JOHN A. MCLAREN
Vice President for Marketing
Evanston Hospital
Evanston, Illinois

CURTIS P. MCLAUGHLIN
Professor
College of Business
Administration
University of North Carolina
Chapel Hill, North Carolina

SUSAN NICHOLS
Assistant Director, Public
Relations
Tennessee Hospital Association
Nashville, Tennessee

RICHARD D. O'HALLARON
Executive Director
St. Mary's Hospital
Richmond, Virginia

THOMAS S. ROBERTSON
Professor
The Wharton School
University of Pittsburgh
Pittsburgh, Pennsylvania

LARRY ROBINSON
Assistant Professor
School of Business
Georgia State University
Atlanta, Georgia

DOUGLASS J. SEAVER
Vice President, Planning &
Operations
Methodist Hospital
Indianapolis, Indiana

JEFFRY STAPLES
Director of Fiscal Services
St. Mary's Hospital
Richmond, Virginia

BARBARA S. TRAEGER
Director of Public Relations
Evanston Hospital
Evanston, Illinois

STEPHEN L. TUCKER
Chairman
Department of Health Care
Administration
Trinity University
San Antonio, Texas

THEODORE R. TYSON
Marketing Consultant
Buffalo Grove, Illinois

M. VENKATESAN
Professor
College of Business
Administration
University of Oregon
Eugene, Oregon

SUSAN WERSHING
Associate Editor
Medical Economics
Oradell, New Jersey

F. BROWN WHITTINGTON
Associate Professor
School of Business
Emory University
Atlanta, Georgia

LAWRENCE H. WORTZEL
Professor
Graduate Program in
Management
Boston University
Boston, Massachusetts

JAY OKUN YEDVAB
Executive Director
Mount Zion Hospital & Medical
Center
San Francisco, California

MINDY ZINN
Project Director, Senior
Citizens Project
St. Clare's Hospital
Community Mental Health
Center
Denville, New Jersey

PREFACE

This assemblage of original, revised, and reprinted works has been drawn together to focus on the context of the new field of health care marketing. The intent is to offer a framework to help practitioners and students of the administration of health delivery systems gain an understanding of the nature and scope of marketing in a health care setting.

It cannot be said that these articles have withstood the test of time and become classics, since health care marketing is a recent phenomenon. In fact, the number of articles from which to choose is limited. Fortunately, as many practitioners have remarked, many of the elements of marketing are not new to the health care setting—they just have not been viewed before in a marketing framework. Consequently, it has been possible to choose from diverse sources. Even though many of the elements have been available, three cornerstones on which the elements of health care marketing could be organized are missing: (1) a framework, (2) a viewpoint, and (3) a definition. Providing these three major components is the objective of this work.

Of the 32 works by 39 authors, ten are written by marketing professionals. Most of the contributions (22) were chosen intentionally because they come from health care professionals. While many of the elements in the framework already existed in the health care literature, there were a few voids that appeared. These voids were filled in three ways: either by original material, by rewritten material, or by introductory comments. Many thanks to Shirley Bonnem, Tony Bushman, Tom Hardy, Dick Ireland, David Karr, Kemsey Mackey, Larry Robinson, Douglass Seaver, and Brown Whittington for their time, effort, and contributions in helping fill those voids. I also am grateful to the other authors and publishers who graciously granted permission to reprint.

A special acknowledgment must be made to Robin MacStravic, who not only provided useful comments as I was developing the concept for this work, but who in many ways is responsible for its existence. It was he who upset the apple cart and created the space for the development of this new field with his book *Marketing Health Care*.

Special thanks go to Mr. Ronald Williams and Ms. Shu-jen Chang. Mr. Williams helped gather material and acted as a sounding board as it was being assembled. Ms. Chang's thoughtful comments and thorough typing helped turn some very rough material into a more comprehensible form. Deep appreciation goes to my wife, Victory, for her patience as I did battle with paper.

While the assistance of others is acknowledged, only I can be held responsible for errors of commission and omission. Articles may have been overlooked because of the diverse area from which this new field draws. New articles undoubtedly will be published. It would be greatly appreciated if any errors or suggestions would be brought to the author's attention so subsequent editions of this collection might clarify ambiguities and reflect expanding viewpoints of health care marketing.

Philip D. Cooper
October 1979

INTRODUCTION

OBJECTIVES OF THE BOOK

Health care marketing is in its embryonic stage. For that reason this cannot be just another collection of readings. If health care marketing were a developed discipline, a readings book would add depth and be a convenience to those reviewing or teaching in the area. The primary objective here is to provide a framework in which the reader can view marketing as it applies to health care delivery systems. Another objective is to draw from the health care literature examples of marketing in today's system with emphasis on administration. Many marketing elements exist already, but until now they have not been united in the health delivery sector. It also has been necessary to develop original material—especially of a conceptual nature—to update previous examples or fill in voids for which suitable readings could not be found. Contributions to this development effort have been made by persons in the marketing and health care fields.

ORGANIZATION OR FRAMEWORK OF THE BOOK

While the emphasis on health care marketing began in earnest in the last half of the 70s, examples from the literature of marketing tools and techniques appeared as early as the mid-60s. What has been missing is a clear understanding of what marketing is and, as a consequence, a focus around which to build a framework. This volume is organized into six basic parts to provide that framework.

The first section lays the groundwork for an understanding of health care marketing and its origins. The first selection, "What Is Health Care Marketing?" is basic and conceptual in nature, while the second, "Consumerism in Health Care Delivery: The Harbinger of Opportunity," focuses on one area—consumerism—and provides examples.

The second major section, "The Marketing Concept: Its Application to Health Care," discusses that concept in the health care industry and its application and acceptance by hospitals. Examples in many of the selections are hospital oriented. This does not imply that health care marketing is the exclusive domain of hospitals. This is far from true. However, most of the available examples in current literature use the hospital as the setting.

The third major section, "Focus on Consumer Orientation in Addition to Nonconsumer Publics," picks up where the selection, "Consumerism in Health Care Delivery: The Harbinger of Opportunity" leaves off. It explores two elements behind the marketing concept. The primary element is consumer orientation because in the past the health care industry—and hospitals in particular—have focused on many of the nonconsumer publics (e.g., physicians; federal, state and local government agencies; suppliers; etc.). While recognition is given to the nonconsumer public, it is not emphasized in the readings selected.

The fourth section, "Health Care Marketing's C.A.P.S.: Specific Areas for Marketing's Contribution," contains descriptions and examples of four major areas where a marketing approach has the potential for the greatest benefit: pricing, how and where services are delivered, development of health services, and promotion. This section, by design, contains a substantial portion of the text. It is the integration of these four areas that provides the backbone for the development of a marketing plan.

The fifth section is "Marketing Research and Marketing Information Systems." The degree to which an organization is committed to the use of marketing research is a measure of its acceptance of the marketing concept. The development of marketing information systems is a form of continuing marketing research. It is highlighted in this section because this volume emphasizes the theme of marketing management as a major input to health care planning. For any plan to succeed it must have controls. Marketing information systems provide such controls.

The last section, "Marketing Plan and Strategy Development," brings all the elements of the book together. The emphasis here is on an overview of marketing in a health care setting and the contributions marketing can make—the integration and pulling together of all functions of a health delivery system, with the common focus on the consumer. The selections contain both original work done for this book as well as material from the literature. The selections provide descriptions of integrative marketing planning and contain many examples, particularly in the hospital setting.

It is hoped that this text will provide an understanding of what health care marketing is and can be.

THE EMERGENCE OF HEALTH CARE MARKETING

OVERVIEW

The impetus for changes in the health care system can be traced back to the consumerism movement. Consumerism will be discussed in the second section, "Consumerism in Health Care Delivery: The Harbinger of Opportunity," by Ray Brown. One of the outgrowths of this movement has been the shift from a "curative" to a more "preventive" approach to health care.[1] Another description of this out growth is the move from "horizontal" or hospital-based care toward "vertical" or ambulatory care. The shift toward vertical care can be seen in the rise of primary care centers in many cities, the resurgence of interest in Health Maintenance Organizations, and government pressure on health care cost containment aimed at the hospital sector in particular.

As noted in the selection titled "Entry Strategies for Marketing in Ambulatory and Other Delivery Systems" (in Section IV), preventive health care is perhaps the easiest and most logical entry point for marketing. Marketing is most easily introduced where the consumer has a high degree of choice. The consumer usually is not forced into preventive health care.

The alarming increase in health care costs in this country has forced society, government, and business to take a hard look at the delivery system. This concern, the resulting emphasis on cost containment, and the changing environment might be interpreted as a crisis for the way health care is delivered now. The Chinese have an interesting way of viewing "crisis." Two characters make up the word "crisis." The first character means "danger," the second, "opportunity." It is the "opportunity" addressed in the second section by Ray Brown.

1

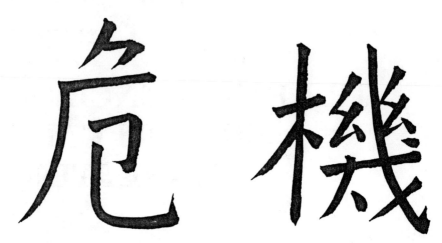

The Chinese characters for "danger" and "opportunity" make up the word "crisis."

First, however, it is necessary to provide a few basic definitions, clarify potential points of misunderstanding and look at the origins for health care marketing. This task is handled by the first selection, "What Is Health Care Marketing?"

NOTE

1. This is pointed out in "The Hospital: Will It Survive?" by Jerold A. Glick, *Hospital Financial Management,* January 1979, pp. 12–18.

1. What Is Health Care Marketing?

PHILIP D. COOPER

While the answer to this question is crucial to understanding the way material is organized in this text, a much broader question needs to be answered: What is marketing? The material by Christopher Lovelock, M. Venkatesan, R. Ireland, and others will provide a number of different answers to this question. For our purposes, a generally accepted and simple definition of marketing is:[1]

> . . . the set of human activities directed at satisfying needs and wants through exchange processes.

The concentration on the issue of exchange is the keystone to this definition, and the focus of the "exchanges" refers to the exchange of "values." These value exchanges can be as simple as the exchange of money for a product or as complex as the exchange of time for a higher level of fulfillment as might be found in participation as a volunteer. Now back to the question: "What Is Health Care Marketing?"

There are two necessary steps that may help to clarify this question. The first step is to provide a definition of health care marketing management. Although some key words in that definition will be described, it is important to clarify the concept upon which health care marketing management is based. Consequently, the second step is to state the basic concepts from which a health systems management philosophy can be derived. While there may be other concepts upon which that philosophy might be based, the three discussed here are the service (product) concept, the selling concept, and the marketing concept.

HEALTH CARE MARKETING MANAGEMENT

Presented below is a philosophy of management that provides a viewpoint that coordinates the operation of both profit and nonprofit oriented health delivery systems.

> *Health Care Marketing Management* is the *process* of understanding the needs and the wants of a *target market*. Its purpose is to provide a viewpoint from which to *integrate* the analysis, planning, implementation (or organization) and control of the health care delivery system.

The output of the health care marketing process is the development of the means to satisfy or facilitate exchanges of values between health care providers and the target market(s).

The words in *bold face* (i.e., process, target market, and integrate) are keys to the full understanding of the definition.

Process

Health care marketing management is a "process," which implies that it is dynamic, not static. The focal point of the "process" is the patient/consumer and certainly the patient/consumer's wants and needs are in a constant state of change. Consequently, a "process" is necessary to keep pace with those changes.

Target Market

While the target market includes a large number of "publics" (e.g., board of trustees, medical and nonmedical staff, community, etc.), it usually refers to the patient/consumer. The accepted description of a user of a health system is a patient. Unfortunately, that label also suggests the way that an individual is expected to behave once within the system. The more active role the individual has been taking in speaking out when things are not right, the development of the Patient Bill of Rights, the increase in malpractice suits, etc., all suggest that perhaps another label might be more appropriate.

The word consumer is introduced here because it has been used by commercial organizations to describe not only those who have been incorporated into the system (or who have become purchasers of products) but also those the organization hopes to attract. Hence, the word consumer has a much broader meaning than patient. The breadth of its meaning is illustrated in Gavin's article titled "Consumer Services: Inhospital Reachout."

Integrate

This is a key word in the definition. Activities that can be described as marketing functions already exist in many areas of health delivery systems. Unfortunately, a philosophy or concept has been lacking that could bring these activities into a coordinated process. It is hoped that health care marketing management, with its focus on patient/consumer satisfaction, can perform this function. One comment made from time to time is that "this (referring to these marketing activities) is nothing new" and has been done for years in hospital or other health care systems. What is new is the integrative approach taken to the various activities to provide a common goal.

In the product-producing sector in the past, as well as today, many firms have operated as a composition of several insulated units. Production was the forbidden ground for sales. It produced the product that then was given to sales to sell or get rid of, as the case might have been. On the other hand, sales departments did not expect production to tell them how to sell. Many other examples (i.e., public relations, accounting, labor relations, etc.) exist. The same phenomenon is true in health delivery systems. The patient comes in contact with several groups that are insulated from each other (office personnel, the bookkeeping department, the provider, the third party payor, etc.) Each group has its own objectives to accomplish.

The marketing concept provides the focus for integrating the efforts of the organization. That focus is consumer satisfaction. As health care delivery in the United States moves away from horizontal care (hospital-based) toward more vertical care (ambulatory facilities), the patient will become a more predominant focus. It is this focusing function that helps to integrate the previously insulated parts of the organization and points out the necessity for planning from a marketing management perspective.

DEVELOPMENT OF A MARKETING MANAGEMENT PHILOSOPHY

Health care marketing management has been defined. It next becomes important to now review alternative viewpoints from which to manage a health delivery system so that the marketing concept might be better understood.

The Service Concept

The first and perhaps the guiding concept that was used as health systems began to evolve was the service concept.

> The *service concept* is the health system's orientation that assumes that the "consumer" (meaning the physician in many instances) will react favorably to good services and facilities and that very little marketing effort is required to obtain sufficient utilization.

The marketing literature and business publications in general make frequent reference to "build a better mousetrap and the world will beat a path to your door." The fallacious assumption is that the product or service stands by itself and is recognized by "consumers" as being superior. It assumes there is no need to design, package, communicate meaningfully to users of the system, select convenient places to distribute the services (or product), or price (referring to monetary price as well as other sacrifices) the service (or product) attractively, etc.

Both profit-making and nonprofit organizations have ascribed to the service concept. The results have been dramatic in some cases. One instance of the failure of the service concept is the classic example of the demise of the railroad industry because it ignored competition's offerings, such as the trucking industry's ability to pick up and deliver door-to-door or the airline's ability to save time. Another example is the performing arts in many cities that produce only the old classics and find audiences and support fading. Health systems are not guaranteed survival by the fact of their existence.

The Selling Concept

This perhaps is more prevalent in the management of profit-making goods than in the health service industry, but it still is a major concept that guides management philosophy.

> The *selling concept* is a management orientation that assumes the system utilizers (physician or patient) will normally not utilize the facilities enough unless they are approached with a substantial selling and promotional effort.

The basic tenet behind this concept is that services are sold, not bought. Insurance and encyclopedia salespersons frequently are used as examples of individuals who feel that the consumer needs to be sought out aggressively. Codes of ethics, common sense, and the disdain for making money off the ills of the public make the application of the selling concept in health systems less than acceptable.

Another tenet is that customers may buy again, but, even if they don't, there are plenty of other customers out there to be sold. There is no great concern about repeat business.

Examples are not limited to profit-making businesses. Nonprofit groups exhibit this concept also. For example, a political party, through the primary process, is provided with a "product" it has to sell. Its sales methodology demonstrates another basic tenet underlying this concept: consumers can be convinced to buy through various sales-stimulating devices (e.g., TV ads, billboard ads, personal selling, giveaways, promises, etc.).

The "selling" of the swine flu program is a good example of the selling concept in action. The government had a service to perform and concentrated on a series of sales-stimulating devices with little regard to the repeat purchase, i.e., future believability in government programs. The result was less than the expected compliance. Indeed, the desire for fast action may have prevented careful consideration of the population's requirement beyond the predetermined medical needs, but some consideration of consumer acceptance could have resulted in a higher level of compliance.

While the selling concept may not be the philosophy behind the operation of various health systems, it has been introduced to help clarify the difference between the selling and marketing concepts. While marketing is gaining prominence in the health care system, many confuse marketing with selling. Consequently, the marketing concept often is dismissed as inappropriate or unethical.

The Marketing Concept

In the commercial business sector, this concept is relatively new. It finds the beginning of its acceptance in the late 50s. The concept basically deals with "exchange" relationships. What follows is an adaptation of the concept to a health systems viewpoint.

> The *marketing concept* is a health system's management orientation that accepts that the key task of the system is to determine the wants, needs and values of a target market(s) and shape the system in such a manner to deliver the desired level of satisfaction.

There are several tenets upon which this concept is based. One is that the system requires an active plan of marketing research to determine what these wants, needs, or values might be. Another tenet is that all the activities that relate either directly or indirectly to the target market (the consumer) must be placed under an integrated marketing control. The material in the last section on marketing planning and strategy (the articles by Ireland, Karr and Seaver) discusses and illustrates what is meant by the need for integrated control. An additional tenet is that if the health care system is successful in satisfying the consumer, the result will be repeat usage, "support" for the system (such as volunteer work, referrals, positive word of mouth, etc.), and consumer loyalty. All these results contribute to the satisfaction of the system's goals.

Exhibit 1 Comparison of Selling and Marketing Concepts

	The selling concept	The marketing concept
Focus on:	The services	"Consumer" needs
Method:	Sole dependence on public relations, health education, etc.	Integrated marketing
Outcome:	Increased revenues through increased usage volume	Increased revenues through consumer satisfaction

The marketing concept is really the antithesis of the selling concept. The selling concept begins with the system's services and believes that through various sales-stimulating devices an acceptable level of usage can be obtained.

The marketing concept begins with existing or potential consumer needs, plans a coordinated set of programs and services to serve those wants, needs, and values, and in return satisfies its goals through creating consumer satisfaction. As Peter Drucker states, "The aim of marketing is to make selling superfluous. The aim of marketing is to know and understand the consumer so well that the product or service fits him and sells itself."[2]

One clear parallel between the focus on consumer needs in the product-producing business sector and the health care sector can be drawn. The difference between "true needs" and the "perception of true needs" is the difference between a marketing and a nonmarketing approach. The product-producing business sector is replete with examples of products that were "perceived" by armchair marketers to meet the needs of the consumers. The classic case of the Edsel is perhaps the best known example. The introduction of the Mustang is the Edsel's antithesis.

Health professionals have long accepted the responsibility for identifying and responding to consumer needs. The predominant practice, however, has been defining needs in terms of how the health professional felt people should behave rather than the actual utilities sought by the consumer or the motivations that influence human behavior. An argument can be made for the value of experience in the field, yet the Edsel also was designed and sold by professionals. It is the focus on the consumer to determine needs that makes marketing different relative to the predominant mode of patient service planning.

THREE SOURCES FOR A MOVE TOWARD HEALTH CARE MARKETING

There are essentially three sources for an organization's changing emphasis to the marketing concept: internal realization, consumerism, and government legislation. Unfortunately, few organizations (private, public, profit or nonprofit) arrive at a marketing concept through internal realization of the value of a true commitment to consumer satisfaction. Organizations as a general rule are reactive to situations. Health care systems are no exception. Health care marketing's development today is due primarily to a combination of consumerism and consumerism's growth into government legislation. No one can argue about the impact of government health care legislation—particularly the Health Service Agency (HSA) and Health Maintenance Organization (HMO) legislation that brings the consumer into the health planning procedure and recognizes the changing need for alternative delivery systems.

Certainly court rulings in many states that have struck down the ban on advertising by professionals, including medical practice, also have opened the door to the judicious use of marketing tools. However, legislation and court rulings do not just happen. Their advent stems from consumerism movements in the 60s. The environment of prosperity allowed the consumer to have greater choice and to seek alternatives. Individuals became more active rather than the passive, patient receivers of relatively scarce goods and services that had typified the 40s and 50s. This rise and its impact on the community hospital sector is chronicled in Ray Brown's article that follows.

NOTES

1. This definition and the concepts of service, selling, and marketing presented later are modifications of material offered in Philip Kotler, *Marketing Management* (3d ed.). (Englewood Cliffs, New Jersey: Prentice-Hall, 1976), Chapter 1.

2. Peter F. Drucker, *Management: Tasks, Responsibilities, Practices* (New York: Harper & Row, Inc., Publishers, 1973), p. 64.

2. Consumerism in Health Care Delivery: The Harbinger of Opportunity

RAY E. BROWN

Adapted with permission to reprint from Duke University Department of Health Administration. The original material appeared as "The Hospital and the Community" in *The Citizenry and the Hospital*, a report of the 1973 annual Forum on Hospital and Health Affairs, Duke University, Durham, North Carolina, Department of Health Administration 27710.

The "community hospital" is an appellation as American as apple pie. It is a term that has been enshrined by hospital public relations people alongside "motherhood" and as a synonym for "compassion," "loving care," and "midnight vigil." It is a metaphor that has guided the deliberations of hospital trustees and the decisions of hospital administrators. The community hospitals of this country entered the decade of the Sixties confident in their belief that they deserved and had won a secure place in the hearts of the communities they were serving. They were little prepared for the infidelity and complications that surfaced during the Sixties within their communities. They were startled by the lack of credibility their metaphor enjoyed.

The decade of the Sixties was one of extreme criticism for all American institutions. Every organized activity in our society was subjected to the new test of relevance by a myriad of diverse new reference groups, and all were given an adverse rating. It was a period that coined a new metaphor of "consumerism." The health care delivery system not only received more of the crescendo of criticism that erupted, but it also felt the censure more. It seemed as if the system were being attacked because of its greatness, and the greater it had become the greater the alienation that had been generated in the hearts and minds of those it served.

The central criticism of the hospital was that it was not responsive to the community. If one examines the record, there is more than a little validity to this criticism. Beneath the rhetoric, and the harsh and unfounded indictments of those who had other axes to grind, there is evidence to support the criticism that the hospital and the medical care system has not looked and listened outside its own walls.

The perspective of the hospital and medical care system has been introverted. It has been so busy keeping in step with medical and technological advances that it has lost step with the community. It has been so preoccupied with what the mailman brought that it has not

11

bothered to see where the mail came from. It has done a tremendous job on the things it has done but it has been much more concerned with the things it was doing than with the needs those things fulfilled. Too little concern has been shown about what ought to be done but an obsessive concern has been exercised about how to do it. Said in another way, the system has given much greater priority to the search for medical solutions than to the quest for community health problems.

Because of the cascading scientific advances, the hospital and medical care system had to run hard to develop the resources, human and hardware, necessary to translate those advances into means for applying them. In doing this it became much more means oriented than ends oriented. It became a fabulous system in terms of its capabilities. Vast programs of research were established to increase and enlarge its technology. Great support was provided for the education and training of doctors and other specialized personnel. Its hospitals became many splendored things. They developed a highly sophisticated set of facilities and staffed them with highly trained personnel. But to the community the hospital and medical care system seemed to become better and better only to serve narrower and narrower ends. Its success seemed to be measured more by the complexity of its resources than by the comprehensiveness of its services. It looked as if the purposes of the system were being organized around its wonderful resources rather than organizing the resources around the appropriate purposes.

Because the system's perspective and posture were inward, the system developed its services to suit the physician and the hospital rather than the community and the patient. The services were organized and provided in terms of what physicians and hospitals decided the community and patients should have, what physicians and hospitals wanted most to do, and what best suited the aspirations of physicians and hospitals. The system set the specifications for its services and asked the community to fit those specifications. It set the conditions under which its services were available and gave the consumer little choice as to how the consumer might be served. It keyed its policies and practices to its own convenience and satisfactions rather than to the convenience and satisfactions of the community it served. It set the boundaries of its services within the doctor's office or the hospital's walls rather than within the best "reach" of the patient. It did not orient itself to serve the patient where the patient was—symptomatically, economically, psychologically, or geographically.

From where the community sat it looked as if its hospital and medical care system had become responsive only to its own expectations. It seemed as if the system had become accountable only to itself.

It would, of course, be highly unfair to say that the hospital and medical care system were the only ones who have not been looking or listening to the community. Actually, whatever looking and listening they did was colored by the reflections of the practices of third parties who stood between the system and the community. The system in a real way had become a captive of the third party financing agencies— both voluntary and governmental. This affected the relationships of the system and the community in two crucial ways. On the one hand it quarantined the influence of the community on the system. The consumer with third party coverage lost his vote because he could not vote with his dollars. He had given his economic proxy to a third party. His community was likewise increasingly voiceless because its hospital increasingly depended upon state-wide and nation-wide third party payors to call the tune.

Because the hospital and medical care system could only have those services and programs that fitted the blanks on third party reimbursement forms, they began to look and listen to third parties rather than to the community. . . . [W]hat the community got was what the system saw on the third party claims form.

All of these factors are not listed as either an indictment or as a defense of the community hospital. Neither is it intended to pass judgment on the overall efficacy and priorities of the services and programs the community hospital has provided its community. Certainly the community hospital has labored hard in behalf of its community. At the same time, however, there has been an increasing disenfranchisement of the community and the individual citizen in the affairs of the community hospital.

One can very validly argue, of course, that the enfranchisement has never been, nor was ever intended to be, very direct or very strong. Historically, community hospitals largely have been owned and operated by local governmental units or by non-profit agencies. The governance of the governmentally owned community hospitals has been the responsibility of the elected representatives of the community and the influence of the individual citizen has been collective and through the polling place. The governance of the non-profit community hospital has been the legal responsibility of its board of trustees. This form of ownership was developed as a deliberate means of removing the hospital from the influence of the polling place. The notion, in both forms of ownership and governance, was that the community was best served if the influence of the individual was subordinated to the processes of government or to the deliberations of a hospital corporate board of trustees.

Legally, the ultimate responsibility of the non-profit hospital trustee is to the institution. He is held accountable for the welfare of the institution and may not put the interests of any individual or any special group ahead of the interests of the institution. This ultimatum has been reinforced numberless times by courts at all levels and in all jurisdictions. This does not mean the interests of the non-profit institution should not be mutual with the interests of those it attempts to serve. Neither does it mean that the trustees should not be alert and concerned with all the needs of the community it serves. It is for this reason that the membership of the board of trustees of the non-profit community hospital should be representative of the varied and diverse interests of its community. That is vastly more than semantically different, however, from saying that a member of the board of trustees should represent special interests groups in the community. To legally and morally fulfill his obligations, the trustee must be capable and free to balance all the legitimate and competing interests of the community.

The excoriation of the "establishment" that is occurring today has fallen heavily on the community hospital. For all the reasons given above, it is quite natural that this is the case. The community hospital has perhaps more disenfranchised the individual citizen than has any other agency or institution in our society. Whether or not the excoriation is a part of the times and will pass away with the times, the community hospital must come to grips with the issue. This is necessary because the hospital has lost its credibility, and perhaps its way.

Providing a voice to the voiceless and hearing the unheard will be no easy thing for the community hospital to do and perhaps cannot be done. Aside from the question of how far can a board of trustees go in sharing its legal and moral accountability, there are other profound issues. On the one hand there is the problem of how much variation and eccentricity the hospital can tolerate in perspective and motivation among decision makers and decision influencers. Then there is the problem of how far professionals can go in sharing their medical and administrative responsibility. Another difficulty lies with the third parties and the difficulties they face in permitting any meaningful influence by varied local groups on programs supported from statewide and nationally derived voluntary and governmental funding. Another problem, paradoxical and perhaps most important, is the acceptance by the community itself of the vagaries of community control. The proliferation of control is indicated only if there is a proliferation of interests or needs to be served. The community hospital is not unique in its inability to go off in diverse directions programmatically and economically at the same time.

The community must coordinate its demands upon the hospital. The hospital's public is a many splintered thing and represents a variety of divergent and competitive interests and goals. No other enterprise is confronted with such great complexity and diversity of relationships. By the nature of its purpose, the intricacy and cruciality of the services it renders, the manner of its financing, its impact on the economy, and its social consequences, the hospital has a heavily pluralistic responsibility. Ambiguity of accountability can only result in conflicting demands on the hospital and getting the hospital into a situation where it is at even greater cross-purposes with the public and with itself.

For these same reasons the community hospital must continuously seek ways and means of becoming more representative of the community and becoming more responsive to the needs and aspirations of segments of the community. It cannot effectively fulfill its role and place in the community unless it is at consensus with the community.

THE MARKETING CONCEPT: ITS APPLICATION TO HEALTH CARE

OVERVIEW

Four articles have been selected for this section. The first two: "Concepts and Strategies for Health Marketers" by C. H. Lovelock and "Preventive Health Care and Marketing: Positive Aspects" by M. Venkatesan are conceptual in nature. They provide supplementary and complementary viewpoints to the material in the previous section on the meaning of marketing and its role in health care. Lovelock looks at health care in general and introduces the notion of competition in health care delivery. Venkatesan addresses the broader concept of marketing and its meaning, but narrows the perspective to preventive health care. This emphasis on preventive care and marketing is appropriate since the consumer is free to choose to use or not use preventive services. This article is divided into two parts. The second part is in Section VI and is titled "Marketing Management–Health Care in General, Preventive Care in Particular" and addresses broader management issues.

The last two articles—"Hospitals Need Marketing Help" by T. R. Tyson and "Marketing As Viewed by Hospital Administrators" by L. M. Robinson and F. B. Whittington—have been chosen because they provide specific examples. The short article by Tyson demonstrates some of the problems many hospitals face plus examples of how hospitals are using marketing today.

The article by Robinson and Whittington summarizes the results of a national survey of hospital administrators. It provides a feeling for the trend toward the use of marketing by describing the types of marketing activities undertaken in the past and charts administrators' opinions about the use of marketing tools and concepts in the next five years.

3. Concepts and Strategies for Health Marketers*

CHRISTOPHER H. LOVELOCK, Ph.D.

Reprinted from *Hospital and Health Services Administration* by Christopher H. Lovelock by the American College of Hospital Administrators, Fall 1977.

Professionals in the health care field are coming to recognize the value of marketing concepts and strategies in helping them do a more effective job of designing and delivering health care services, and of developing and implementing health education programs. But despite the interest in marketing, it is often misperceived and misused. Clarification of key marketing concepts and their strategic implications may provide helpful guidelines for health care marketers.

Many people equate marketing with advertising and selling. Actually the field is much broader. It's often divided into four major elements known as the *Marketing Mix,* namely (1) Product, (2) Price, (3) Distribution, and (4) Communications. Advertising, selling and public relations are simply part of the communications element of the mix.

The Concepts of Product and Exchange

Marketers use the word product in a generic sense to denote what is being offered in the marketplace. It could be a physical good such as toothpaste or a new drug, or a service such as a haircut, X-ray or eye-refraction. Alternatively, it might be something as intangible as a politician offering a political platform, a college offering an education, or an agency holding out the promise of better health through improved nutrition.

Central to marketing is the concept of exchange—consumers giving something in exchange for the product. While money is the most common quid pro quo, time and other personal variables may also constitute part of the exchange transaction.

Pricing Considerations

In those situations where products are sold rather than given away, and there is a dollar price attached, purchasing decisions may be influ-

---

*Paper prepared for presentation at conference on "The Responsibility of Hospitals to Educate for Health," sponsored by the American College of Hospital Administrators and the Academy of Hospital Public Relations, in Philadelphia, April 29–30, 1976.

enced not only by the level of price charged, in dollars and cents, but also by how the price may be paid: Are all transactions strictly cash or are checks and credit cards accepted? Are credit terms offered and, if so, what are they?

However, there may be other sorts of costs incurred by the individual in addition to financial ones; these may include time and inconvenience as well as the psychic costs associated with changing established values and behavior patterns with which the individual feels comfortable, overcoming personal fears or risking social disapproval by others. Sometimes people are reluctant to use a product or service which is offered free of charge or to adopt new behavior patterns because the non-dollar costs outweigh the apparent benefits.

Distribution

The selection of a distribution strategy—the place where the product is available—may be a very significant factor in determining a marketer's success or failure. Often consumers can obtain similar products or services from a variety of different retail outlets. The choice of a particular retail outlet may be made as much on the basis of the convenience of the location, the appearance and atmosphere of the facility, and the helpfulness and expertise of the sales staff, as on the extent, quality and value of the merchandise or services sold there.

Proximity of customers to the source of a service can affect both demand for the service and the degree of satisfaction with it. Consumer analysis has often led to the relocation of sources of services closer to users' locations. For example, government agencies providing social and welfare services utilized primarily by low income or elderly groups are increasingly thinking in terms of locating their offices in or near the neighborhood in which these people live rather than downtown. Bus routes which were established years ago are now being re-routed to take into account new travel patterns resulting from changing home, shopping and employment locations.

Hospitals, especially older ones, are often located in deteriorating central city locations with limited parking. This may serve to discourage use by middle income people who have moved out to the suburbs where newer, more attractive and more conveniently located competitors may be found. Since it may not be desirable or feasible to move the building, marketing strategies for dealing with this situation might include developing outside clinics in locations near target consumers, provision of improved access (e.g., institution of a shuttle bus service from a suitable parking lot elsewhere), or construction of parking facilities providing safe, direct access to the hospital buildings.

The Role of Communications

Communications policy is a critical ingredient in virtually all marketing programs. Even a well-designed product or service, intended to satisfy a demonstrable consumer need, is unlikely to achieve much success unless target consumers (1) are aware that it exists, (2) understand what it is supposed to do for them, and (3) have at least some idea of where and how to obtain and use it.

Note that I have described communications as "a critical ingredient" in marketing. All too many times, nonbusiness marketers take product, price and place as given, viewing advertising, personal communications, and various publicity activities as the only ingredients in a marketing program. Let me suggest a set of questions which those responsible for marketing communications ought to be asking themselves so that a consistent overall marketing program can be developed, using each element of the marketing mix:

Questions for Marketers

- What are we marketing? In other words, what is our product and what does it offer various segments of the population? Is the nature of the present product appropriate and, if not, how might it be changed?
- To whom are we marketing it? Sometimes a product is intended for one and all. Alternatively, certain segments of the population are targeted for special attention. Does the product meet the needs of those groups to whom it is primarily directed? Are some important groups being overlooked?
- How are we marketing it? What role (if any) does pricing play in the marketing program and how was a price arrived at? Does it take into account the price-sensitivities of target consumer groups? Additionally, what communications are we using to inform people of the product and to encourage them to use it? Are the messages employed appropriate for these target groups? Are efforts made to reduce psychic costs?
- Where are we marketing it? This speaks to distribution issues, notably physical location and how convenient it is for the target segment(s). However, it can also include concerns relating to the physical characteristics of the facilities themselves. Are they comfortable, cheerful, properly heated and cooled? The same question can also extend to the locations in which communications messages are distributed—are these locations where the target consumers are likely to hear or see them?

- When are we marketing it? Is the product or service available on a 24-hour basis, seven days a week, or only for limited periods? If the latter, are these likely to be the most appropriate times of the day/week for the target segments? A weekday morning clinic is probably less convenient for working men and women than an evening or weekend one would be, unless it is easy for them to get time off work without loss of pay. Timing considerations are also significant in scheduling messages in the broadcast and print media, with a view to maximizing the chance of reaching target consumers at a time when they are not only likely to be exposed to the message but also attentive towards it.

Health care marketers are often placed in a difficult position in that decisions relating to the nature and quality of services offered, as well as when and where these are offered, and how pricing policy is set, are not always perceived as being within the province of marketing. Again, this suggests a very narrow view of what marketing's role really is.

This leads to a final question which may seem obvious but often isn't. Why are we marketing this product? In the business sector, the long-run objective inevitably centers around profitability. For nonprofit and public organizations, where profits are not the name of the game, the mission or objectives are likely to vary widely. Unless this mission is properly articulated and appropriate measures of performance developed, it is very difficult to formulate a marketing strategy; strategy requires clearly established objectives and a means of subsequently measuring how well these objectives have been met.

The Notion of Competition

Marketing activities are usually concerned with people's behavior, either seeking to change it or reinforce it. One toothpaste manufacturer may urge us to buy his brand, while another may seek to woo us away from established brands by introducing a new brand with yet another miracle ingredient. It's easy to recognize the presence and implications of competition in such a situation.

Hospitals or clinics may be reluctant to admit that they are in competition with one another, but within certain limits they often are, offering similar services at similar prices to the same range of prospective patients who might as readily travel to Hospital X as to Hospital Y.

It may be harder to conceptualize the nature of competition for public health education. However, it does exist and failure to recognize the fact may result in an ineffectual marketing campaign.

Such competition may take several forms. The most obvious is a direct, frontal attack by an opposing organization on the program being marketed. Anti-fluoridation, anti-abortion and anti-birth control campaigns are an example. Sometimes campaigns of this ilk are undertaken for sincere reasons by groups with strong beliefs and values; sometimes there are sound medical reasons for questioning the use of particular medications (e.g., birth control pills) or health practices. Programs of opposition may represent expressions of political beliefs or simply the views of the "lunatic fringe."

It is a moot point when to counter competing communications of this nature and when to ignore them rather than drawing further attention to them. Sometimes, opposition reflects genuine defects in the position (product) advocated by the public health agency (in which case it should be corrected forthwith); alternatively, opponents may simply misunderstand the product, in which case new communications may be needed to correct these misperceptions. In both instances, some marketing research at the outset might have yielded a better initial marketing program which avoided such problems.

Countering the Competition

A major problem arises when health programs advocating a change in behavior, such as anti-smoking, anti-alcoholism and anti-drug abuse, must compete with the promotional activities of tobacco, liquor and barbiturate manufacturers or the personal urgings of friends, acquaintances and professional "pushers." In such situations, lobbying for legislative controls or "equal time" may be an appropriate strategy.

Perhaps the most subtle form of competition to health education programs designed to change behavior lies within individuals themselves. It is easier to reinforce existing behavior than to change it. Change may be disruptive of present habits or it may simply be an effort for the individual. Here we return to the notion of non-financial costs—time, inconvenience, and psychic costs. Woe betide the marketer who overlooks them!

Flossing one's teeth properly is time-consuming and a nuisance; so is fastening safety-belts, which may connote a sissy image as well as restricting freedom of movement within the vehicle. Nutritious food may, especially initially, look and taste less attractive than so-called "junk foods." Giving up smoking or drinking may induce withdrawal pangs. Taking more exercise is tiring and time-consuming—and initially may make you feel awful; much pleasanter by far to relax with a six-pack in front of the television. Going for hypertension screening may seem scary to some, take time, and involve travel and expense; the immediate outcome may be that you learn something unpleasant about your health at the end of it all. Inoculations are painful, sometimes costly, and also take time and effort.

Proper use of medications requires a level of precision and regularity which conflicts with some people's vague, easygoing lifestyles. Some authorities believe that self breast examination is suffused with fear and emotion for some women. Practicing birth control is contrary to many people's values. The list is almost endless, since matters of health and safety are so intimately related to how we live our daily lives.

What the New Behavior Costs

In every instance, there is a perceived "cost" associated with the recommended new behavior which outweighs the benefits (if any) which the individual anticipates receiving as a result. The need for public health marketers to understand the nature and origin of such costs cannot be overemphasized. This may necessitate consumer research.

In many instances, marketing strategies can be developed to neutralize or at least minimize the impact of such competitive forces. Clinical treatments can be made less threatening by conducting them in a relaxed, friendly environment; mobile units can reduce the need for travel to a central location; new inoculation techniques (or simply better training of those who inoculate) may make such experiences almost painless; substitute approaches, such as use of air-bags, may achieve safety belts' benefits at less bother to the consumer; improved communications may clarify benefits, simplify required changes in behavior, and perhaps reiterate possible negative outcomes of noncompliance in ways which are meaningful to the consumer and provide added motivation for change.

However, different groups of people require different approaches. Individuals differ from one another in both physical and mental characteristics, they live in different places and are exposed to different media. So-called mass communication campaigns designed to appeal to all often end by influencing no one. Instead of thinking of mass markets, public health markets need to consider the opportunities for market segmentation.

Market Segmentation

In evaluating a market and developing appropriate programs, one of three broad alternative strategies can be followed. The first is market aggregation in which all consumers are treated alike and a single marketing program is developed for everyone.

Many broad-based public health programs fall into this category. While such an approach promises considerable economies of scale, it often loses effectiveness as a result of its failure to recognize the varying needs, concerns and behavior patterns of different groups within the population.

At the opposite end of the scale is total market disaggregation where each consumer is treated uniquely. In the last analysis, each individual may be thought of as a separate market segment on the grounds that each person is slightly different from everybody else in personal characteristics, behavior patterns, needs, values and attitudes.

Good personal medical care may fall into this second category, with the practitioner developing a tailored program of treatment for each patient, offering personal advice and instructions, possibly charging according to ability to pay and, in the "good old days," often being willing to make house calls rather than insisting that patients come to the doctor's office.

When developing educational programs for health, however, complete individualization may be too time-consuming and costly. This is where the third approach, market segmentation, has much to offer. This calls for grouping consumers with certain definable characteristics in common. Marketing programs can then be developed which are tailored to each group.

The concept of market segmentation is based upon the propositions that (1) consumers are different; (2) differences in consumers are related to differences in market behavior; and (3) segments of consumers can be isolated within the overall market. A number of benefits may result from adopting a segmentation approach, including:

- a more precise definition of the market in terms of the needs of specific groups, why they behave as they do, and possible ways of influencing behavior;
- a better ability to identify competitive strengths and weaknesses, and opportunities for winning specific segments from the competition;
- more efficient allocation of limited resources to development of programs which will satisfy the needs of target segments;

- clarification of objectives and definition of performance standards.

The basic problem is to select segmentation variables which are likely to prove useful in a specific operational context. Three criteria must be satisfied if meaningful market segments are to be developed:

1. Measurability: it must be possible to obtain information on the specific characteristics of interest.
2. Accessibility: management must be able to identify chosen segments within the overall market and effectively focus marketing efforts on these segments.
3. Substantiality: the segments must be large enough (and/or sufficiently important) to merit the time and cost of separate attention.

Segmenting the Market for Health Education

Three basic categories of market segmentation are usually proposed in marketing, each capable of subdivision into a variety of separate variables: geographic, demographic, and psychographic.

1. Geographic segmentation groups people by the locations where they live, work or regularly visit. There is generally a limit to how far most people will travel for non-specialist, ambulatory health care and marketing programs should realistically be focussed on that segment of the population which enjoys easy access to the facility. Emphasizing the word *access* implies that time and ease of travel is often more significant than actual mileage. In a broader context, such as a national or statewide public health program, it is important to recognize differences in health needs by region, reflecting variables such as climate, pollution levels, quality of water supplies, etc. Communications programs should take into account the coverage of different media—billboards are obviously very location-specific, but there are also geographic limits to the circulation of particular newspapers and to the transmission range of radio and TV stations.
2. Demographics are probably the most commonly used set of segmentation variables for health care marketing. Age and sex are obviously related to health care needs, as may be such readily identifiable physical characteristics as height and weight.

Some ethnic groups are more prone to certain health problems than others (e.g., sickle-cell anemia); other implications of ethnicity may include dietary habits and difficulty in understanding English; some religions have dietary prescriptions and strongly influence attitudes towards certain health-related practices. Differences in income levels often have implications for nutrition as well as for ability to pay for medical care. Educational level — sometimes highly correlated with income — is often associated with understanding hygiene, attitude towards medical treatment, and ability to understand the need for specific behavioral changes. Frequently, demographic characteristics such as income, ethnicity, age and education are closely associated with geographic location, reflecting the tendency of different demographic groups to form homogeneous clusters in clearly defined neighborhoods. Census data can often be valuable in clarifying the demographic characteristics of areas as small as a city block.

3. Psychographic segmentation refers to the lifestyle, attitudes and behavior patterns of individuals. People within the same demographic group often exhibit vast differences in these characteristics. Lifestyles, eating and drinking habits, working conditions, awareness of and attitudes towards health issues, past medical history, current state of health, self-image, personal beliefs, fears, and emotions — each of these can play a significant role in determining an individual's needs for health care, receptiveness to health-related communications, willingness to adopt new behavior patterns and specific benefits sought.

After reviewing several studies, one researcher concluded that consumer behavior in the health care field was shaped more closely by psychographic factors than by demographic ones.[1] Unfortunately, psychographic variables are often the hardest to identify, making it difficult to seek out and reach such segments with services and messages tailored to their specific situations.

It is more difficult to practice market segmentation strategies when the target segment is not clearly identifiable within the general population. For instance, a health care program may be developed to treat hypertension, clinics sited in what are believed to be appropriate locations, and a flexible pricing policy established. However, informing those who could benefit from the treatment in question and persuading them to use it may be difficult. In such instances it may be necessary to use wide-area media targeted toward the segment for whom it is intended. Additionally, referral strategies can be developed whereby the message is passed down through intermediaries, such as employers, who may even be able to provide screening facilities.

Conclusion

It is very important to recognize that advertising, public relations and personal communications constitute only one category within the broader marketing mix. Each of the other elements in this mix plays a role in determining the success or failure of the overall program. It's not merely a matter of looking at all the elements in the mix, but also of ensuring that they mutually reinforce each other to produce an internally consistent program.

Success is also a function of the marketer's ability to understand the different needs, attitudes, characteristics and behavior patterns of the various segments that make up the mass market, and then develop programs tailored to these segments. In many instances, this will pose a need for market research, both as an input to planning and as a means of monitoring subsequent performance so that appropriate modifications can be made for the future.

What I want to argue for strongly is involvement of marketing specialists from the outset in formulation of any health program directed at educating or caring for members of the public. All too often, it is only after a program or service has already been developed that someone with marketing skills is called in and instructed to "tell people about this," or "urge them to do such and such." In many instances, even that is frowned upon in the health care field. Indeed, it is only recently that certain institutional taboos against advertising in the medical profession have begun to be challenged.

Even though such prohibitions may not apply to the field of public health education, institutional prejudices die hard and there may still be resistance to giving marketing professionals any significant responsibilities outside a limited and strictly reactive communications role.

What this suggests is *a need to market marketing itself to health care professionals,* highlighting the discipline's responsiveness to consumers and clearly defining what it can and cannot do. Just as undesirable as blind resistance to marketing is the unrealistic expectation that marketing can be the salvation of the health care industry.

NOTE

1. Lawrence H. Wortzel, "The Behavior of the Health Care Consumer: A Selective Review" in B. B. Anderson (ed.) *Advances in Consumer Research, Vol. III* (Association for Consumer Research, 1976).

4. Preventive Health Care and Marketing: Positive Aspects

M. VENKATESAN

Reprinted from *Marketing and Preventive Health Care*, pp. 12–25, Cooper, P.D. et. al. eds., by permission of the American Marketing Association, Chicago, Illinois, 1978.

There is increasing emphasis and focus on prevention of serious illnesses or accidents rather than repairing the damage after the fact. During his campaign, Jimmy Carter advocated that

> prevention is both cheaper and simpler than cure, but we have stressed the latter and have ignored to an increasing degree the former. In recent years, we have spent 40 cents out of every health dollar on hospitalization. In effect we've made the hospital the first line of defense instead of the last. By contrast we've spent only three cents on disease prevention and control, less than one-half a cent on health education and one-quarter of a cent on environmental health research.[1]

There is now increasing emphasis on prevention of every kind—medical, occupational, environmental and nutritional.

It is believed that significant improvements in health can be made through changes in life style. Marketing is looked upon as one avenue to affect the life style area. Increasingly, there is recognition that marketing can play a vital role in the whole range of health care services offered in our society. Recently Evanston Hospital in Evanston, Illinois created a position of "vice president marketing" and it is believed to be the first such appointment at any hospital.[2] Other commercial marketing practices such as special promotions and advertising to make potential consumers aware of some of their services are also being adopted by hospitals. For example, the Sunrise Hospital at Las Vegas, in an attempt to spread the incoming patient-load evenly, is offering prizes ("once in a life cruise") and Skokie Valley Community Hospital is engaged in an advertising campaign to make the community aware of its alcoholic treatment center.[2] Hospitals have not escaped problems similar to corporations in terms of their names, logo and the like. An example is illustrated by problems of recognition and comprehension created by the change of name of the University of Iowa hospitals from

"Iowa Regional Health Care Center" to "Iowa's Tertiary Health Care Center." One of the reporters for the *Des Moines Register* who interviewed a nonscientific sample of patients of the facility found that among consumers "tertiary" had no obvious connection to medicine or health care![3] It may be obvious that increasing marketing intrusion in the health care area may be timely, unavoidable and may even be necessary for the survival of the health care industry. Even the troubling experiences of the newly created HMOs attest to the lack of marketing knowledge and expertise in introducing these new concepts in the health care area. As Ellwood aptly observed, "Marketing has been a forbidden field for the health professional. With the exception of health insurers, marketing skills and knowhow are in short supply."[4] It is in this context that this paper attempts to present a view of how marketing can play an important role in the offering of health care services for prevention.

Confusions and Misconceptions

Confusions and misconceptions abound about the term "preventive health" and "marketing." The confusing state of affairs results from lack of any delineation as to what the term preventive health includes. Depending on the writer and on the occasion, it includes everything from jogging, flossing of one's teeth, inoculations for children, to early detection of cancer, heart disease and the like and the range extends to wearing safety belts and changing the life style of the individuals radically by redesigning the urban environment.

Misconceptions about marketing, its role and functions stem from the lack of awareness of the macro and micro aspects of marketing. Most of the writers point to educational campaigns and advertising efforts in such areas as family planning, mass immunizations, seat belt usage and the like to point out that marketing does not work. There seems to be little recognition or realization that the advertising or selling function (as emphasized in HMO enrollment schemes) is *not* marketing—at best, they constitute a single element of marketing instruments conventionally employed by business firms.

The second type of misconception or misunderstanding stems from the view that marketing is really catering to "artificially created demands" or that while it may be necessary to market products such as shampoo, cereals and automobiles, it is not necessary to market health. One writer in the health area has asserted (in a denial of consumer choice process and sovereignty) that "the problem in the health area is not how to give people what they want, but how to change people so that they will want what *we* have to offer. To be more precise, physicians decide what is good for people to do and people are expected to do it."[5] Some others would have governmental agencies banish certain products[6] or ban commercials on the television programs (and in print medium too)[7] in order to promote preventive health measures! Such suggestions reflect little faith in the intelligence of the masses whose welfare is presumably at the heart of these suggestions! Finally, some of the misconceptions are the result of excesses and abuses by Madison Avenue and in the marketing of some products and services by some unscrupulous organizations.

There is very little awareness, understanding or appreciation of the enormous amount of activities carried out under the bailiwick of marketing management and the relevance of these commercial marketing management activities to health care areas. The important point to recognize is that marketing is a process and is performed in both profit and nonprofit making organizations. Marketing management has reached very sophisticated levels and it utilizes highly refined research tools and concepts. Thus the inescapable conclusion is that the health care area may very well benefit immensely by the use of demonstrated marketing management concepts, tools and methods. . . .

What Is Marketing?

Marketing should be viewed as an *exchange process*. As in any exchange, it involves two or more parties, each with something to exchange. The parties should be able to communicate what they are exchanging and to be able to deliver to consummate the exchange. Thus, marketing is defined "as the set of human activities directed at facilitating and consummating exchanges."[8] The desired exchange relationships do not come about naturally or automatically. They require skillful planning and management of the process. As such, marketing management is defined as follows:

> the analysis, planning and implementation, and control of programs designed to bring about desired exchanges with target audiences for the purpose of personal or mutual gain. It relies heavily on the adaptation and coordination of product, price, promotion and place for achieving effective response.[8]

Viewed in this framework much of what goes under the category of marketing in the health care services in general and preventive services in particular is but one element of marketing. (e.g., educational or persuasive advertising alone is used many times with very little marketing strategy involved in the efforts).

There are two aspects of marketing—one dealing with macro aspects which relate to aggregate problems largely beyond the control of an individual organization. The impact of technology on changing existing products or changes in the production processes and products resulting from technological changes or the impact of legal environment on marketing practices in the economy are all illustrations of the macro aspects of marketing. These are usually treated as "uncontrollable variables" from the viewpoint of an individual organization. The second aspect of marketing which is concerned directly with the operations of an individual organization are the micro aspects of marketing. Stated differently, the firm or any organization has control only on certain marketing variables such as product, price, communication (promotion), and place (logistics). The planning, directing and controlling of these "controllable variables" often called the "marketing mix," are the basic tasks of marketing management.

Marketing Concept

The present day marketing concept views marketing as a social process, the purpose of which is the identification of consumer wants and the satisfaction of these wants through integrated marketing activities.[8] Such an orientation removes the traditional view of marketing as simply moving goods from production to consumption. Thus marketing must focus on the needs of the buyer and not be preoccupied with seller's needs. Some view growth of consumerism and criticism of marketing practices as resulting from the failure of many firms to adopt a consumer orientation in their marketing activities.

It is well to remember this marketing concept of consumer orientation as we embark upon marketing management's relevance to preventive health care activities. For, as the following observations vividly illustrate, preventive health care providers seem very much [in] the tradition of "sales orientation":

> The kinds and amounts of goods and services produced and offered in the commercial market are usually adapted to consumer demand. No competent entrepreneur will produce or try to sell goods unless he has reason to believe that there is already a substantial demand for them. Moreover he will package, offer and distribute them in ways that he believes will attract the attention of people who are already interested in his type of product and to make the product appear as one that best fits existing demands for such goods.

In contrast, the health actions on which we try to "sell" the public are given. They are defined relatively exactly and inflexibly by the health practices, whether preventive or therapeutic, can be and are only to a very limited extent tailored to consumers' desires, motives or preferences. In fact, many and perhaps most of the actions we would like consumers to take are inherently unpleasant, inconvenient, humiliating, painful, or disruptive of cherished living habits. There is precious little we can do, to fit the product to the consumer's taste, to package it attractively, or to make it otherwise more palatable.[5]

Even the present HMOs view their marketing function as involving simply an enrollment activity—a selling activity, which is usually planned for after all other organizational plans are completed. . . .

REFERENCES

1. *Wall Street Journal,* February 24, 1977, p. 20.

2. *Wall Street Journal,* March 24, 1977, p. 1.

3. *Des Moines* (Iowa) *Register,* March 4, 1977, p. 1.

4. Ellwood, Paul M., Jr., and Michael E. Herbert, "Health Care: Should Industry Buy It or Sell It?" *Harvard Business Review,* July-August, 1973, pp. 99–107.

5. Hochbaum, Godfrey M., "Selling Health to the Public," in *Consumer Behavior in the Health Marketplace.* Editor: Ian M. Newman, Nebraska Center for Health Education, University of Nebraska, Lincoln, Nebraska, pp. 5–14.

6. Robertson, Leon S. "Whose Behavior in What Health Market Place?" in *Consumer Behavior in the Health Marketplace.* Editor: Ian M. Newman, Nebraska Center for Health Education, University of Nebraska, Lincoln, Nebraska, pp. 5–14.

7. McKinlay, J. B. "A Case for Refocusing Upstream: The Political Economy of Illness," pp. 7–17.

8. Kotler, Philip, *Marketing Management,* Second Edition, Prentice-Hall, Englewood Cliffs, New Jersey, 1972.

5. Hospitals Need Marketing Help

THEODORE R. TYSON

Reprinted from *Advertising Age,* pp. 65–66, by permission of Crain Communications, Inc., ©
February 13, 1978.

The health care industry is in trouble. Hospitals, the biggest and
most visible segment of the industry, are in the most trouble.

In a peculiar and contradictory fashion, hospitals are simultaneously
condemned both for what they do, and what they don't do. In any given
week, hospitals will be castigated by legislators, consumer advocates
and the media for:

1. Having too many beds—or not enough beds.
2. Making money from the sick—or losing money through poor
   management.
3. Employing too many people—or [providing] poor service because of insufficient personnel.
4. Buying unnecessary costly equipment—or not having the
   latest lifesaving equipment.

The "experts" will now rush in and state unequivocally that other
industries have been subjected to the same treatment and handled it
smartly because they ran their business in a more efficient way.

There's no denying that a hospital is a business that sells its products to customers and, like any business, it can always be operated
more efficiently. But unlike most businesses, it operates in a mode and
environment that the average business would find untenable, if not
downright impossible. For example:

1. Not only is the "product" (treatment for illness) not really
   wanted by consumers, but its purchase is seldom planned because one can't predict appendicitis, pneumonia, heart attacks
   or kidney failure.
2. The hospital's "salesmen" (doctors) who bring in the "customers" (patients) are not employed by, controlled by or paid by the
   "company" (hospital).
3. Customers can't shop for "suppliers" (hospitals) in the conven-
   tional sense and find it difficult to make a price-value comparison of the products that are available.
4. Over 70 percent of the "company's" (hospital's) customers do
   not pay for the product themselves; rather, payment is made by

35

"third parties" (Blue Cross, Medicare, etc.) who do not use the product—but tell the hospital how much they will pay, when they will pay and under what conditions they will pay.

In addition, the accelerating cost of hospitalization (acute in-patient care) has put hospitals under tremendous pressure to modify the traditional health delivery system by introducing new and expanded programs that emphasize preventive medicine and out-patient treatment.

This means that for the first time hospitals must communicate directly with their various consumer segments, not merely in the classic public relations sense, but for the acceptance and purchase of their new "products." The combination of a deteriorating image, a unique set of business problems and a mandate to change direction has led hospital executives to seek new methods of evaluating the viability of services and communicating with different market segments.

Recently professionals in health care have come to recognize the practical value of marketing in the development of strategies and tactics that will more effectively deliver health care services. With increasing regularity, articles that define and exemplify the use of marketing are appearing in leading hospital publications such as *Hospitals, Modern Healthcare, Hospital Progress* and *Hospital and Health Services Administration.*

Seminars and workshops on marketing health care services have been conducted, or are planned, by such august organizations as the American College of Hospital Administrators, the American Hospital Association, the Academy of Hospital Public Relations, the American Marketing Association, the Wharton School and Northwestern University.

Most importantly, marketing is being used today at the grass roots hospital level. Here are some of the ways:

1. A major teaching medical center is developing a marketing plan to sell contract management services to smaller hospitals.
2. A 600-bed community hospital is using market evaluation and marketing planning to help construct the most effective strategy for its long-range plan.
3. A 230-bed community hospital is using market research to assess its position relative to competitive institutions and to determine what current and future services its various market segments need, want and will utilize.

However, the use of marketing by hospitals is still in its infancy and its misuse can adversely affect the health of an already troubled hospital system. What hospitals don't need is slick marketing designed to:

1. Fill hospital beds, thereby exacerbating the already unacceptable cost of health care.
2. Promulgate the utilization of unnecessary services, further reducing the public's confidence.

What hospitals do need is help from marketing professionals who will take the time to learn the hospitals' problems and products.

The hospital industry is a sleeping giant, awakening to the use of marketing. With revenues of $64 billion and 35,000,000 customers, it's a market you can't afford to ignore.

6. Marketing as Viewed by Hospital Administrators

LARRY M. ROBINSON AND F. BROWN WHITTINGTON

There is a rapidly growing literature on the subject of health care marketing. In fact, one bibliography contains, in annotated form, some 226 entries, more than half of which were authorized between 1976 and 1978.[1] A review of the literature shows considerable differences with respect to both definitions and acceptance of health care marketing. However, one point is clear. There is intense interest on the part of health care professionals to develop an increased understanding of marketing. This reading addresses possible reasons for the emergence of that interest, considers some of the issues debated in the literature, reviews the results of a nationwide survey of hospital administrators on the use of marketing techniques, and examines implications of the survey findings.

HEALTH CARE MARKETING: AN AWAKENING OF INTEREST

Exhibit 1 suggests reasons for the emergence of interest in health care marketing. The list was developed from a class discussion in a graduate course on "Marketing for Health Services Organizations" at the Medical School at Emory University in Atlanta. It summarizes some of the external forces that constrain health care administrators and that require effective response. The public, through elected officials, has required greater accountability from providers of health care services. Administrators also are faced by increased levels of competition for the opportunity to meet the health care needs of the community. In addition, health care consumers have changed substantially in recent years. Their expectations have increased and many have broadened their understanding of available options.

Other reasons for emergence of health care marketing have been suggested. Berkowitz and Flexner, in a review of three earlier articles, stated:[2]

> Some potential benefits (of health care marketing) include: increased capacity to respond to the needs and wants of consumers, personnel and the community in general; classification in the development of long-range strategies and objec-

Exhibit 1 Some Reasons for Rising Levels of Interest in Health Care
Marketing

Reason	Explanation
1. Rising costs	With rapid escalation of health care costs has come a search for methods and techniques to slow the rate of increase. Marketing may be useful to health care administrators in effecting cost containment measures.
2. Rising accountability	Legislation has created mechanisms for review of health care service providers. Providers are now required to have information to support requests for additional services and to defend the allocation of resources. Marketing techniques and concepts are useful in the development of such information.
3. Trustees and directors have placed increasing emphasis on the health care consumer's needs	Administrators must demonstrate to governing boards that health care consumers have been consulted and their needs considered in planning and operating the services offered.
4. Increase in proprietary health care services	There have been widely reported successes of such profit-making health care services as hospital management firms, proprietary hospitals, health maintenance organizations, group practices, and emergency clinics. As a result, many health care organizations believe that they must become more competitive and devote increased attention to their principal markets.
5. Underutilization viewed as waste	Marketing provides the administration with concepts and techniques to smooth irregular demand patterns, to review consumer needs, to identify and reach target markets, and to measure customer satisfaction with services offered. Thus, marketing may be useful in increasing levels of utilization without creating demand for unneeded services.
6. Duplication of services	Marketing can assist administrators to measure total demand, assess the level and quality of services offered by other health care providers, and determine which services should be offered to meet effectively the needs of the markets served by the organi-

Reason	Explanation
	zation. Thus, marketing can provide information to assist decision makers in their quest to achieve effective utilization of available financial, human, and equipment resources.
7. Rising sense of professionalism by staff	Increasingly, nurses, pharmacists, respiratory therapists and other staff members seek recognition for their contributions. Marketing, with its emphasis on exchange relationships with key publics, provides an approach to administrators faced with an increasingly complex set of staff needs and expectations.
8. Changing nature of patient-physician relationship	Patients have become more active participants in decisions affecting their health care. Choices with respect to where, how, and what health care services are sought are influenced increasingly by consumer awareness and knowledge. Marketing techniques are useful in development of consumer awareness and in providing information about alternative services.
9. Rising interest in prevention	While most consumers still seek health care on an episodic, curative crisis basis, there is a clear trend toward utilization of preventive health services. Preventive health services possess characteristics that are amenable to marketing efforts, and that can reduce the overall costs of health care substantially.
10. Rising consumer dissatisfaction with health care providers	Expectation levels of health care consumers are rising. Therefore, health care providers must develop better understanding of consumer expectations and satisfaction levels. Marketing provides the measurement techniques needed to determine patient expectation and satisfaction.
11. Health care as a business	Many observers believe that health care possesses the elements of a business. That is, there are products and services that are offered to consumers by competitors at prices and locations that differ substantially. Effective public relations and promotional techniques also use the same principles as do business firms.

tives; and more effective allocation of resources within the organization.

The points raised by these authors were reinforced in the June 1, 1977, issue of *Hospitals* in six articles on hospital marketing. The editors presented the articles with the comment that ". . . hospitals no longer can afford to assume they know what their communities need."[3] Marketing, with its focus on determination of consumer needs, was viewed as being useful to hospital administrators.

Some hospital administrators have embraced marketing for defensive, perhaps even survival, reasons. MacStravic, in two articles, has referred to "efforts to limit and even reduce the supply of hospital beds," and[4] "to the reduction in what third party payers will pay for, and to increasing pressure from review agencies to limit inpatient services."[5] In addition, McLaren noted that "Some hospitals are moving toward marketing because of lagging patient admissions . . . to strengthen referral patterns . . . (or) because they are planning to expand their physical plant."[6]

Marketing has become a topic of intense interest to health care administrators. John Alexander McMahon, president of the American Hospital Association, wrote that:[7]

> The mention of hospital marketing brings a reaction from almost everyone. Some positive, saying it's the wave of the future; some negative saying it will undermine the voluntary hospital system. And both views often are supported equally well.

This statement summarizes the often emotional debate over the utility of marketing in the health care sector. Next, some of the points often raised in the debate over health care marketing.

ISSUES IN HEALTH CARE MARKETING

Exhibit 2 provides an overview of points in favor of, and in opposition to, the use of marketing by health care providers. Supporters of marketing believe it can help administrators to define changing consumer needs, assist in the development of needed services, attract consumers with the needs, and then satisfy the identified needs with a product or service at the quality and price desired. In fact, as management authority Peter Drucker has noted, effective marketing occurs when the product or service meets consumer needs so well that no selling effort is required.

Exhibit 2 Issues in Health Care Marketing

Pro	Con
Marketing is more than advertising, selling, and public relations. It includes all activities required to plan, facilitate, and conduct voluntary exchanges to mutual benefit. Health care marketing is a process of determining what health care consumers need, tailoring services to meet those needs, and then attracting patients to use these services.	Marketing is the same thing as advertising. Marketing is the same thing as selling. Marketing is the same thing as public relations. Marketing is equated with "hucksterism" and manipulation.
Health care marketing recognizes that health care is a service with differentiable characteristics. Marketing techniques reduce the cost of health care by helping consumers and providers to make more rational and efficient decisions.	Active competition may force health care providers to promote, thus increasing the cost of health care to the community. To label health care a "product" is ultimately to demean it.
Health care organizations must become competitive in a variety of markets just to survive.	Active competition may lead to unnecessary utilization.
Competition is an inescapable reality. Without competition, there is little incentive for efficient and effective utilization of scarce resources.	Hospitals should not promote and expand services at the expense of other hospitals. Competition could cause hospitals to focus on filling beds rather than on providing needed services. Given extraordinary regulations that health care to which providers are subject, a true market orientation probably is not possible.
Marketing is value free. It is a set of concepts and techniques that can be used for good or for evil.	The misapplication of marketing methods can damage the service reputations of health care institutions.
It is legitimate to position a hospital as the one in the community that provides only routine inpatient services, and to thus establish a lower daily service charge than hospitals with highly specialized services.	Hospitals will be affected adversely by competitors who become known as "discount health care stores."

Critics of health care marketing, on the other hand, note that use of marketing may increase demand for unnecessary services while lowering the quality and service image of the health care system. Cutthroat competition also could be ruinous to some institutions, resulting in lowered availability of quality medical care.

It would appear that both critics and advocates have overstated the power of marketing as applied to health care. However, it is clear that marketing is being used effectively by a small and growing number of health care organizations. Yet little or no empirical evidence exists on the extent and nature of present and anticipated uses of marketing by hospital administrators. Accordingly, a study was conducted to answer these and other questions:

1. What marketing practices are carried out now by U.S. hospitals?
2. What marketing concepts and practices are perceived by health care professionals as appropriate for hospitals?
3. What are the perceptions of health care professionals for the future of marketing in hospitals?

Methodology

A total of 350 hospitals, stratified by geographic region and number association, was sampled. A mail questionnaire sent to the hospital administrator at each institution produced 191 responses, for a response rate of 54.6 percent. Highlights of the study follow.

Does Marketing by Hospitals Exist Today?

The study asked administrators if their hospital carried out (or planned for) 11 selected marketing-related activities. Their responses are summarized in Table 1. Examination of this table provides several interesting insights.

Marketing Research Activities Are Practiced by a Substantial Proportion of Hospitals

These activities, including definition of target markets, patient attitude surveys, and study of competitors, apparently are acceptable to the hospital community. Perhaps they are acceptable because hospital administrators do not attach a marketing concept label to them. Also, with the exception of patient attitude surveys, these marketing research efforts can be performed discreetly with no infringement on personal privacy. In addition, each of these activities is an initial step in meeting competition from local institutions. The activities probably are not used as an integrated plan but will be moving toward formalization in the future, as evidenced in the next section.

Hospitals Rarely Practice Formal Marketing Planning, but a Substantial Increase in Such Planning Is Expected

Few administrators indicated they now used a formal marketing plan. Possible explanations for this low use may include: (1) the recent advent of the use of marketing tools in the health care environment; (2) the apparent lack of clear methodologies for establishing formal marketing programs; and (3) the apparent undesirable connotation to administrators of the term "marketing." More than twice as many hospitals planned to initiate a formal marketing program as those that had programs at the time of the survey. This increase may have indicated that administrators recognized that marketing activities should be integrated into a formal plan.

Few Hospitals Bestow "Marketing Title" on a Staff Member

Administrators who responded appeared to be saying that the term "marketing" may invoke an unfavorable image in the minds of the community and, perhaps more importantly, physicians. However, the administrators also may be saying that the marketing function in a hospital setting has not matured enough to warrant a person's carrying a title such as Associate Administrator–Marketing. Respondents indicated there would be little increase in the number of administrators with a marketing title in the future.

Patient-Oriented Advertising Was Used in a Substantial Number of Hospitals

Historically, hospital administrators have viewed their institutions as professional subunits of the physician. Since the American Medical Association discouraged advertising by physicians, the typical hospital also avoided advertising. However, the data suggest a growing acceptance of advertising by hospitals. The data are consistent with the posture of the American Hospital Association, which in August 1977 published *Guidelines for Advertising by Hospitals*. The guidelines encourage advertising to promote awareness and to provide information on unique or distinctive service offerings.

What Activities Should a Hospital's Marketing Program Include?

A second part of the questionnaire asked hospital administrators to indicate which of 11 marketing activities should be included in a hospi-

Table 1 Respondents' Opinions of Marketing Activity To Be Included in a Hospital's Program

Activity	No. of hospitals responding to this question	Percent Responding				
		Certainly should be included	Probably should be included	No opinion	Probably should not be included	Certainly should not be included
Attitude survey of current or discharged patients	181	87	13	0	0	0
Marketing research techniques to assist in feasibility studies	182	45	41	12	2	0
Patient-oriented advertising	182	21	31	15	26	8
Direct mail promotion to physicians	183	39	26	10	20	5

Patient demographic profile	179	73	15	11	0	1
Staff member with well-defined marketing responsibilities	181	28	42	21	6	3
Defined hospitals target market	182	71	18	10	0	1
Formal marketing plan	180	38	37	19	3	2
Seminars for medical professionals	182	70	24	5	1	0
Study of services offered by nearby hospitals	182	81	16	2	1	0
Lounges for physicians	182	71	18	9	2	0

NOTE: Totals may not add to 100 percent because of rounding.

tal's marketing program. These responses are summarized in Table 1. These data were compared with the "present practice" responses in Table 2 to provide further information on the status of hospital marketing.

Most of the Marketing Activities Listed Were Perceived to be a Desirable Part of the Hospital's Program

Several of these activities probably were being used already by the respondent's hospital. Only two activities—patient-oriented advertising and direct mail promotion to physicians—did not enjoy more than a 70 percent positive response rate. In fact, all 11 activities were favored by more than half of the respondents.

Respondents Strongly Favored a Staff Member with Well-Defined Marketing Responsibilities

The respondents also indicated that a formal marketing plan was a desirable feature. These findings suggest a positive future for marketing in hospitals. It would appear that marketing activities may be coordinated by an administrator for marketing operating under policies established in a formal marketing plan.

Patient-Oriented Advertising and Direct Mail Promotion to Physicians were the Most Likely Candidates for Omission from a Marketing Program

Before sounding a permanent death knell, one must recognize that these promotional activities have been repugnant to health care professionals in the past, but with the advent of recent Supreme Court decisions on advertising by professionals and the increasing pressure for high occupancy, an increase in its acceptability may be forthcoming.

The Future of Marketing by Hospitals

A third section of the questionnaire requested opinions about seven factors affecting the future of marketing by hospitals. These responses are summarized in Table 3.

Marketing Was Perceived as a Legitimate Function of Hospitals

This positive perception by a substantial proportion of administrators should be encouraging to the marketing discipline. It also pre-

Table 2 Marketing Activities of Hospitals Affiliated with the American Hospital Association

Activity	No. of hospitals responding to this question	% of respondents carrying out this activity in 1977	% of respondents planning this activity for future
Attitude survey of current or discharged patients	181	70	8
Marketing research techniques to assist in feasibility studies	176	34	5
Patient-oriented advertising	181	20	8
Direct mail promotion to physicians	180	39	6
Developed patient demographic profile	184	46	17
Had staff member with marketing in job title	183	4	4
Defined hospital's target market	179	59	18
Implemented formal marketing plan	182	9	19
Seminars at hospital for medical professionals	181	71	7
Study of services offered by nearby hospitals	180	64	10
Lounges for physicians	176	77	9

Table 3 Respondents' Opinions of Factors Affecting the Future of Marketing by Hospitals

Statement	No. of hospitals responding to this question	Percent Responding				
		Strongly agree	Mildly agree	No opinion	Mildly disagree	Strongly disagree
Marketing is a legitimate function of hospitals	182	58	32	4	3	3
Marketing activities by hospitals will increase in the next five years	182	68	24	6	2	0
Our hospital can carry out marketing functions more effectively if the term "marketing" is avoided	182	26	44	20	8	2

Hospitals should promote themselves and their activities	183	78	15	1	4	3
Sufficient detailed problems are available for effective hospital marketing	181	14	31	18	27	10
Our staff of physicians strongly supports a formal marketing plan	182	7	27	40	19	7
Our board strongly supports a formal marketing plan	179	13	32	38	12	5

sents a formidable challenge to develop techniques that will be of special use for hospitals. Further, marketing professionals should be active in expanding the perceptions administrators have of the contributions marketing activities can provide to successful management decisions.

An Increase in Marketing Activities by Hospitals Was Forecast

Such a projection presents a further challenge to marketing professionals. Before hospital marketing can expand significantly, the value of such activities must be made apparent. The proverb "nothing succeeds like success" is appropriate here because successful marketing activities should encourage hospital administrators to broaden their usage of marketing activities.

The Term "Marketing" Hinders the Implementation of the Function in Hospitals

Apparently as long as marketing activities are not called "marketing activities," they will continue to enjoy growth of legitimacy and usage. A much better job of "marketing marketing" to hospitals must be done to erase the prevalent image of hucksterism. Hospital marketers must accept the challenge to share successes with their peers through journals, speeches at professional meetings, and seminars devoted to the proper application of marketing concepts in the hospital setting.

Promotion of Hospitals and Their Activities Was Seen as Desirable

The highly favorable response to the concept of promoting hospitals and their activities may seem inconsistent with the unfavorable responses to questions on promotional activities. The answer to this apparent inconsistency may be that administrators wanted the community and physicians to know the activities in which the hospital was involved but administrators did not believe that patient-oriented advertising and direct mail promotions to physicians were appropriate means. Perhaps an expanded use of publicity, to inform key publics of progress and new services, would be more consistent with accepted hospital administrative practice.

Administrators Disagreed on the Sufficiency of Available Marketing Procedures

The responses may indicate an unequal distribution of detailed information about marketing. On the other hand, many administrators may have been unaware of the existence of appropriate marketing information. Further, the state of the art of hospital marketing may be so young that a truly useful set of marketing procedures has not been developed.

Conclusions

Hospital administrators' diagnoses of hospital marketing were favorable. Most marketing functions were in use or were planned for implementation. The term "marketing" was not used by hospital administrators to give an umbrella description to marketing activities. Administrators generally believed that most marketing activities about which they were questioned should be included in a hospital's program.

The prognosis for marketing in hospitals also was favorable; but with several caveats. Administrators saw marketing as a legitimate hospital function, but were uncertain about the proper use of advertising. Marketing professionals should respond to these views by focusing on the particular hospital problems that marketing activities could help solve. Those interested in hospital marketing also should devote considerable effort to show administrators the positive uses of marketing techniques.

Administrators definitely believed that the use of marketing activities by hospitals would expand. To determine the success of marketing, professionals should develop evaluative criteria that will help hospitals measure their success. Administrators expressed a desire to promote the hospital and its activities, but viewed promotion activities used by businesses as unprofessional and unacceptable. Professionals should seek methods of tasteful and ethical promotional methods to meet the needs of both the institution and the community it serves.

Clearly, more work of a theoretical and practical nature must be done. There exists an excellent opportunity for the academic community and hospital practitioners to work together in developing new dimensions for the marketing and health care professions. The authors share the view expressed by Cooper and Kehoe in their summary of a workshop on health care marketing held at the 1978 Educators' Conference of the American Marketing Association:[8]

> The marketing and health care professions stand on an exciting threshold. In ten years it is hoped that the integration will be fully operationalized. The end product will be of a symbolic nature and ensuing benefits will accrue (in a marketing con-

cept view) to the focal point of both the health care professional and the marketer—the health care consumer.

NOTES

1. Larry M. Robinson and Philip D. Cooper, "Health Care Marketing: An Annotated Bibliography." Unpublished manuscript. Atlanta: Georgia State University, January 1979.

2. Eric N. Berkowitz and William A. Flexner, "The Marketing Audit: A Tool for Health Service Organizations," *Health Care Management Review,* Fall 1978, pp. 51–57.

3. "Should We Market Health Care?" *Hospitals,* 51 (June 1, 1977), p. 51.

4. Robin MacStravic, "Marketing Health Care Services: The Challenger of Primary Care," *Health Care Management Review,* Summer 1977, pp. 9–14.

5. _____ , "Should Hospitals Market?" *Health Progress,* August 1977, pp. 56–59, 82.

6. John A. McLaren, "Marketing Assures a Satellite Facility a Safe Sendoff," *Hospitals,* 51 (June 1, 1977), pp. 67–69.

7. American Hospital Association, *First Quarter Report 1977,* pp. 1–8.

8. Philip D. Cooper and William J. Kehoe, "Health Care Marketing: An Idea Whose Time Has Come," *Proceedings of the 1978 Educators' Conference of the American Marketing Association.* (Chicago: American Marketing Association), pp. 369–372.

SECTION III

FOCUS ON CONSUMER ORIENTATION AND NONCONSUMER PUBLICS

OVERVIEW

In the past, emphasis has been placed on physicians, suppliers, political groups, etc. by health delivery systems (hospitals in particular) but a shift to a consumer-oriented philosophy has been occurring. The article by Ray Brown in Section I is a good introduction to this section. The events in the hospital sector during the 60s led to "A Patient's Bill of Rights" approved by the American Hospital Association House of Delegates in February 1973. These actions and others have set the stage for the shift in focus and orientation to the consumer.

The first article, by Tim Garton, blends the consumer and nonconsumer focus. The author discusses the benefits of creating a good image and the understanding of constituent groups as the basis for design of hospital services. He also raises the issue of marketing's place in a system of National Health Insurance. The second article, by Yedvab, explores consumer involvement and satisfaction, the key role of the administrator, and the inputs and organization needed to help with the job of developing consumer orientation.

The next three articles provide specific examples of the use of consumer orientation. All three focus on the hospital as the forum for expressing marketing's consumer orientation. Stephen Tucker views the exchange relationship between the hospital and two of its "publics" (i.e., the patient and the medical staff members) and discusses the needs of these publics and how the hospital can satisfy them. The article by Cassidy and Constantine and the original article by Shirley

Bonnem concentrate on how specific hospitals focus on the consumer. The Bonnem article goes a step further by looking at how a children's hospital determined the needs of the physician public and how a Long Island hospital met the needs of the "community at large" public.

7. Marketing Health Care: Its Untapped Potential

TIM GARTON

Reprinted, with permission, from *Hospital Progress*, February 1978. Copyright 1978 by The Catholic Hospital Association.

The health care field is often accused of madly rushing off after whatever is new or timely. Today, the concept of marketing health care services has suddenly become a topic of great interest among administrators. People who arrange meetings are planning discussions of it, entrepreneurial academicians are rushing to prepare two-day seminars to teach all one needs to know about marketing, and the professional journals are opening space to this previously taboo subject. Marketing is being heralded as something new and exciting—a challenge that the enlightened administration must rise to meet. Still, with all of this activity and interest, the health care industry has not yet considered the full implication of adopting a marketing orientation for health care institutions.

Marketing has long been recognized as a legitimate management function by virtually all for-profit institutions worldwide. Yet due to a long-standing misunderstanding of the marketing function, eleemosynary, or nonprofit, institutions have shied away from its use. One reason for this lack of concern about marketing is found in the origin of most hospitals in this country. Hospitals have tended to emerge in response to an easily identifiable demand, usually from a broad spectrum of society. From their founding, hospitals sought to include direct community input through the linkages between identifiable community groups and resources and the board of trustees.[1]

As the size of the industry and of individual institutions grew, the desires and needs of the community and the nature of the constituencies the hospital served became more fragmented. No longer are a hospital's constituencies' needs easily identifiable. Thus, for the future, the promise that marketing holds for hospitals seems all the more desirable.

Marketing smacks of Madison Avenue. It brings to mind mass media promotional campaigns and the thought of millions of dollars invested in the name of brand-differentiating competition. All of these ideas seem foreign to an industry the ideals of which revolve around humanitarian service to the community. Consequently, for years marketing has been ignored because it was viewed as unethical. Finally, those involved in training hospital administrators have also ignored marketing as a subject until recently. Thus, most practicing administrators were not exposed while in school to the formal techniques and often complex technologies of marketing.

For these basic reasons, marketing has never been recognized as a legitimate part of hospital administration; and though indications are that this is changing, the question remains, Is marketing a legitimate part of the health care business? . . .

What Marketing Promises Hospitals

Marketing concepts and techniques properly applied can have wide-reaching positive effects for a hospital. The promises of marketing can be categorized as contributing to the creation of a unified image, to the development of a better understanding of constituent groups and their demands on the hospital, or to the appropriate design and promotion of the hospital's services.

Throughout all contacts and across the widespread differences in orientations among groups, the hospital's image should remain constant. Corporate image campaigns are growing in acceptance among major multiproduct diversified organizations. Traditionally, these campaigns focused on the use of mass media to develop an awareness of the company's name and product lines. For a hospital, however, the concept of presenting a unified public image extends well beyond simple advertising. It includes all relationships the hospital enters, whether with employees, physicians, community leaders, governmental or regulatory agencies, or the patients themselves. The image that the hospital chooses to present must be equally clear to those affiliated with the hospital (employees, trustees, volunteers, physicians, and others) and to those who are not directly affiliated with the hospital.

Many hospitals have an established image. Most do not. Usually the image of the hospital differs depending on which group of perceivers one considers. Employees may feel that the organization is rigid and inflexible and that as a result the quality of care suffers. Suppliers may think of a hospital as an average customer, while physicians think it the best place in town. What the public's opinion would be under these circumstances is anyone's guess. Establishing a pervasive, uniformly favorable image for the hospital is imperative if recruiting, development, and government relations efforts are to be successful.

Hospitals generally have a very strong geographic identification. As a result, presenting a unified image could attract a wide spectrum of the population in the immediate area, but it could also alienate certain portions. Thus, the image a hospital should seek to promote is one of steadfastly meaningful service to the entire community.

In order to effectively meet the needs of the community, a hospital must first determine the size, nature, and orientation of all of the hospital's publics. This research and subsequent market segmentation is the second major marketing function of hospitals. In consumer products marketing, a great deal of effort has been spent in developing effective methodologies for developing profiles of the individuals that will purchase certain types of products. Research is aimed at identifying these individuals (for a hospital, a patient origin study), the factors that weighed heavily in their decision to buy (for a hospital, such items as location, physician preference, quality of food, "homelike" atmosphere), and those among this group who were presented with the opportunity to buy one product but bought another (e.g., people from the hospital's immediate service area who bypass the hospital in favor of care elsewhere). Any promotional effort is totally dependent on this evaluative stage. Only by determining the basic demographic and life style characteristics of the community the hospital serves can the organization focus on the needs and demands of particular segments.

Market segmentation is simply the process of identifying subgroups in the population the hospital serves that have similar needs, demands, interests, orientations, or resources that directly affect their decisions to seek certain services from the institution. I have argued that it is important for the hospital to discover what the community thinks about the institution as a whole. It is equally important that the hospital know how young married women feel about the obstetrics program at the hospital. Hospitals are able to target their services based on fundamental principles of public health or epidemiology, but thus far, they have not been similarly able to target their investigation of the community's reaction to individual services or to the range of services provided.

Finally, the use of marketing techniques and concepts promises the hospital aid in developing new services, in properly positioning the hospital's services in relation to the alternatives available, and in effectively promoting the services to various targeted groups. Despite some claims otherwise, competition between hospitals exists, most often competition for inpatients. Some persons say this is unimportant, since it is only at the margins; but realizing the difference a 5 percent increase in occupancy can have in the financial health of the hospital and in its ability to generate new programs points to the importance of effectively presenting the hospital to its publics. Marketing techniques developed in other industries can help the hospital place its services in the most favorable light and, thereby, maximize its services to the community.

Briefly, these are the promises marketing makes to a hospital: a more unified image, a better understanding of constituent groups, and an appropriate design and promotion of the hospital services.

Changed Orientation Is Marketing's Challenge

In order to effectively use marketing techniques, a hospital must change its very orientation, shifting its emphasis from products toward people. Traditionally, hospitals have sought to provide a basic set of services and to improve them over time. With each technological development, hospital services became more sophisticated and less understandable to the layperson. Thus, the gap in knowledge between professionals and the patients they served grew. Because the field was advancing so rapidly, providers began to focus on the services and the products they produced and to ignore the total effects on the ultimate consumer, the patient. Studies have traced the decline in perceived physician "bedside manner" to the explosion of medical knowledge in the 1950s.[1] The lack of meaningful communication between doctors and patients, however, is only the tip of the iceberg.

Institutions blinded themselves to many of the needs of patients during the 1950s and early 1960s. Resources were seldom expended with the aim of facilitating the patient's access to certain services. Rather, the hospital spent its time and resources on the tremendous rise in technological competence in health care. Only in the last 10 years have the institutions begun to consider the overall effect that policies and procedures can have on patients, employees, and physicians. This is partly reaction to labor organizing activities, younger physicians' militancy, more patient complaints about lack of dignity, and a much stronger patient propensity for litigation. One of the first signs that administrators were becoming more responsive to patients was the increased use of functional design principles for patient rooms. For the first time, the industry became concerned with the dignity of the patient—from the patient's viewpoint, not from that of the providers.[5] Change has been slow, but it has been accelerated by the increased militancy of consumers and the spread of distrust of technology and professionals that seems to have begun 10 years ago. Recently, Rick Carlson and Ivan Illich have lambasted the medical field for its strict product orientation.[6] While they clearly overstate the problem, their ideas lead to the fundamental challenge posed by the adoption of marketing techniques: Do the people really know what they want? And the corollary: Is what they want what they need?

Adopting the attitude that the hospital's constituents are aware of their desires or demands allows the organization to approach each group from a different perspective. This is the essence of market segmentation.

One major constituent group is the medical staff. Proprietary hospitals have long utilized a host of marketing techniques to encourage community-based physicians to admit patients to their facilities. Yet how much does the average hospital know, in a systematic way, about the orientation of its medical staff? Generally, all a board of trustees or a senior administrator sees is a consensus, such as a desire for new machinery or capital expenditures. Seldom are they truly aware of the underlying orientation of each physician, which is so important to the institution. Where physicians have multiple appointments, understanding the needs or just plain preferences of the consulting or courtesy staff members could cause a few to admit another patient or two to the facility. In the aggregate this could be a significant contribution to occupancy. Beginning simply, one might ask each physician what would make the hospital a more attractive place to practice. For many institutions the answers could be quite revealing.

Asking that question assumes physicians actually know what they really want. That isn't too difficult a concession to make. But if the question is posed to patients instead of to physicians, assuming that patients know what they want requires a new outlook for many institutions.

The use of promotional techniques is designed to alter the perceptions of individuals and thereby affect the utilization behaviors. This does not, however, obviate considering patients' desires and being willing to modify services accordingly. Certainly one can produce persuasive appeals without regard to the constituents' desires, but therein lies the difference between good and bad marketing programs.

Marketing's Role in Consumer Education

Marketing is an important management tool for all hospitals. It demands a new orientation and promises growth in the institutions' ability to meet the needs of the community and to bring the individuals in their areas to a greater awareness of what medical care can offer. Research on consumer behavior—that is, on the decision to purchase—could hold the key to a longstanding health care problem: How can health behavior be influenced? In the past the field has relied exclusively on the concept of implied rationality. That is, anyone would prefer not to smoke if shown a nonsmoker's pink lung next to a heavy smoker's dirty black lung. The plain truth is that these mass media promotional programs based on fear and the rational framework of some nonsmokers have failed. And despite cross-sectional studies, it really is not known why some people seek physicians' care, while others don't.[7] Moreover, the ability to directly affect health behaviors, such as smoking, drinking, diet, exercise, is minimal. If a hospital is involved in community health education, then it may be forced to look outside the traditional community education programs to the more sophisticated and meaningful approach that good market research can bring.

Inappropriate utilization of hospital resources by the community has plagued hospitals for years. One reason it persists may be that the public is relatively ill informed about the nature of the services provided or about how to use them properly. The public would be better off if better informed; and marketing can play the key role in providing people with information they can use and with the encouragement to use it.

Marketing Requires Expertise

Marketing poorly applied can be a disaster for the hospital and a terrible waste of community resources. It can be just as much a disaster as would be a poorly designed building or poor financial management. The need for training in the use of marketing concepts and principles is apparent. Today qualified, capable people are lacking in the field. A few academicians, well trained in marketing, have "dabbled" in the health field; but too often they have made fundamental errors in data interpretation because they are not familiar with the intricacies of professional and institutional interrelationships in this field.

For example, I read a study done by two young marketing researchers. They produced excellent instruments to gather data, ran an appropriate set of controls on the data gathering, and produced a superior set of information. Based on their data, however, they concluded Health Maintenance Organizations were sweeping the country. Their interpretation of the data was completely fallacious, and the excellent scientific work was meaningless. Thus, while many of the basic principles of marketing can be directly applied to the hospital, others simply cannot be so applied. Many academics new to the health care field are unable to discern which principles fall into which of these categories.

Administrators, consultants, and physicians have attempted to apply some marketing principles to hospitals, but most of these persons are not sufficiently aware of how to use market research techniques. On the other hand, a few consultants are qualified and capable of using these techniques, and a large number of administrators have been using them for years but calling them something else, usually planning.

While marketing as a discipline is new to the health care field, it has used marketing concepts for many years. All successful institutions have the pieces of a good marketing program, but they have not combined them into as effective a tool as possible. Some authors have suggested the solution that hospitals organize for marketing by establishing a marketing department and acquiring capable people to run it, usually from other industries.[8] But why should people from other industries be successful in the health care field?

For the larger urban hospitals and especially for hospital groups or consortia, an effective ongoing program requires organizational development. For the smaller community hospital, this is not justified. In the latter situation, the administrator or one of the senior assistants can easily assume the responsibility for combining the talents of others in the organization to develop an effective marketing program, once this individual has studied the discipline with the same fervor with which such a person might approach financial management.

Simply stated, the problem of health care marketing is that those in the field have ignored marketing. Can they expect to add this management tool immediately or with little effort? Or can they reasonably expect people not trained in the health care field to be able to make the application for them? They tried the wholesale importation of management talent from other industries in the late 1960s. Perhaps the industry has progressed beyond that strategy.

Marketing principles and techniques must be aggressively considered by current administrators. Those who are at all interested in marketing must make sure they are well informed. But that is not an easy task. Marketing is a developing field. Few people are adequately trained in both health administration and marketing. Thus, until their number and influence grow, hospitals must approach the use of marketing cautiously.

Certain Techniques To Be Carefully Avoided

... The hospital industry's ability to advance its own political fortunes depends in large part on its ability to generate and maintain a meaningful consensus among the institutions. The field may appear fragmented because large and small institutions or urban and rural institutions or proprietary and nonprofits can't get together. The overly aggressive use of marketing techniques could foster resentment among different organizations and destroy whatever spirit of cooperation exists. In the face of growing government involvement in planning the health care system, hospitals can ill afford to appear callous to the development of an integrated medical care delivery system.

Marketing for hospitals can and must be unobtrusive. Its purpose is to facilitate the hospital's efforts to meet the community's needs. It must not appear as an attempt to manipulate the community for the benefit of the institution.

Marketing is not always successful in business, as it is highly dependent on the product delivered. If advertising raises expectations above the ability of the product to satisfy, it will destroy that product. Perhaps people will be enticed to try it once, but then the product's future is dismal. Hospitals are in the community for the long haul. Raising inappropriate expectations (the health care field has always been guilty of that) is bad marketing. It is an attempt to manipulate the community, and ultimately the community will know this. Abuse of this kind is the difference between ill-advised and well-planned uses of marketing.

One question remains to be tackled. If the nation had a universal, compulsory national health insurance program, would hospitals be as concerned about marketing as they are now? In one sense, I think they would. Marketing can aid in disseminating appropriate information about using the health care system and also can try to provide the persuasive link between change in knowledge and change in behavior.

This is an issue with which hospitals have struggled for years. Inappropriate utilization of emergency departments remains an unsolved problem. Abuses of the system, primarily the result of ignorance, abound. There is little continuity of care in many organized ambulatory care settings, partly because patients don't understand the system. And patients don't always fit into the system. A flexible marketing orientation is necessary to accurately assess the structure of programs, to initiate changes as they seem appropriate, and to use promotional techniques to encourage patients to adapt to the system where that seems most appropriate.

Introducing a comprehensive national health insurance program, especially one with increased emphasis on organized ambulatory care and the use of paraprofessional medical personnel, will only exacerbate these problems. But, the system can use marketing techniques to inform the community about the practical results of changes in coverage, privileges, and services available. Without a unified, meaningful flow of information, the community could be completely confused for years, thereby hampering effective utilization of the system's resources. Marketing, therefore, could hold the key to the effective introduction and implementation of a national health insurance program.

On the other hand, marketing can be viewed as an investment in the competition between hospitals. Hospitals serve relatively defined service areas. At the edges, or margins, of these service areas there is friction or competition between hospitals. Direct benefits result from investing in this competition today; but will that be true when and if the third party payments are all standardized?

NHI Could Intensify Ethical Issues

Viewing the question from this angle sharpens the focus on ethical issues. Is it acceptable for a health institution to expend community resources to increase its power, dominance, or influence by increasing the inpatient census when that may cause another institution to decline? Many influential people in the field feel quite strongly that hospitals should not use precious resources to devour each other. They feel that there is little room for divisive competitive promotion today and that under a universal set of revenue and reimbursement controls, a hospital promoting itself would be definitely out of place.

Yet, if one takes the view that national health insurance will likely not wipe out the private-paying prerogative in the United States, then marketing could become extremely important to the individual institutions. The situation could evolve into one very similar to that currently found in the long-term care industry, where the vast majority of patients are covered by poorly paying Medicaid programs and the nursing homes stiffly compete for a minority of private-paying patients. If a nursing home fills about 20 percent of its beds with private-paying patients, it is successful; with less than 5 percent of these patients, its survival is tenuous. Hospitals might find themselves in a similar situation under a national health insurance program. Relative success in attracting private-paying patients could be the major determinant of whether an institution would be able to initiate and support innovative or specialized services. It could be the major determinant of a hospital's autonomy. Thus, investment in marketing could become significant under a national health insurance program.

The need for caution remains. Under any system marketing techniques can and probably will be abused. Just as there are a few overly zealous construction management firms, there may be some overuse or outright abuse of marketing principles. The solution lies in cautious moderation. Conscious attempts to manipulate the consumer's decision to purchase health care are new to the health care field. The direction they should take is not easily determined.

Marketing is a neutral instrument. An institution's simply adopting marketing techniques does not commit it to Madison Avenue styled promotional campaigns. It simply indicates its willingness to adapt the products and services of the institution to the needs and desires of the organization's constituents. Other industries have spent years and millions of dollars on the perfecting of basic techniques of data gathering, data analysis, market segmentation, advertising research, and a host of other tools that the hospital too can use. These tools can be used by the hospital to better meet the needs of the community.

This discussion has emphasized the use of marketing to discover the needs and desires of the community served by the institution and to meet these needs and desires. When properly conceived and directed, marketing is most certainly a part of the health care business.

NOTES

1. Jeffery Pfeffer, "Size, Composition, and Function of Hospital Boards of Directors: A Study of Organization-Environment Linkage," *Administrative Science Quarterly,* September 1973.

2. Philip Kotler, "A Generic Concept of Marketing," *Journal of Marketing,* April 1972.

3. J. F. Engel, O. T. Kollat, and R. D. Blackwell, *Consumer Behavior,* Holt, New York City, 1973.

4. See, for example, Milton Davis, "Variations in Patients' Compliance with Doctor's Advice: An Empirical Analysis of Patterns of Communications," *American Journal of Public Health,* February 1968; or Gerry Stimson, "Obeying Doctor's Orders: A View from the Other Side," *Social Science and Medicine,* February 1974.

5. Leon C. Pullen, "Nursing Unit Design," mimeograph available from Herman Smith Associates, Hinsdale, IL, 1970.

6. Rick Carlson, *The End of Medicine,* Wiley, New York City, 1975; Ivan Illich, *Medical Nemesis,* Calder and Boyars, Ltd., London, 1975.

7. R. Andersen, J. Kravits, O. Anderson, *Equity in Health Services,* Ballinger, Cambridge, MA, 1976.

8. See, for instance, Richard O'Hallaron, Jeffry Staples, and Paul Chiampa, "Marketing Your Hospital," *Hospital Progress,* December 1976.

8. Consumer's Role in Defining Goals, Structures, and Services

JAY OKUN YEDVAB

Reprinted, with permission, from *Hospital Progress*, April 1974. Copyright 1974 by The Catholic Hospital Association.

The concept of the consumer's role in health care is in a constant state of flux and crisis, and this state will probably continue for a long time to come. A basic ground for misunderstanding is the assumption that the term "consumer" has a universal meaning.

An individual's perspective affects his definition of and approach to the health care consumer. A hospital administrator identifies consumers as current and potential patients in his own hospital, as the individuals residing in his hospital's geographic neighborhood or service area, and as the physicians who comprise the hospital's medical staff. To the administrator, the latter are both consumer and provider. A physician identifies consumers as his own patients and those of other physicians.

A hospital trustee conceives of consumers as those individuals for whom he shares the legal and moral responsibility to provide care. More particularly, he thinks of those individuals for whom care is actually being provided at the hospital on whose board he serves. More generally, he must consider those individuals who donate to the hospital, and, if he serves on the board of a sectarian-sponsored facility, he must consider the hospital's sponsoring community.

A hospital controller probably defines the consumer by adding the number of dollars the hospital collected during a specific year divided by the number of patients who paid all or part of their bills, plus the number of third-party payers who paid the remainder.

To a congressman, state legislator, or local politician, a consumer is anyone in his own district who either can or will be able to vote and who has needed or may need health care.

Yet no matter how we define consumer, we must pay attention to consumer advocates such as Ralph Nader and Herbert Dennenberg, who are raising serious questions about the health care system. They have no solutions, but they are raising relevant questions. Whoever consumers are, they include the government, employers, and labor unions — any organization that offers benefit plans. In fact, corporations and large unions with their multi-million-dollar health and welfare programs rank next to government as the biggest consumer of health care.

The International Brotherhood of Teamsters has declared that the California Council for Health Plan Alternatives (a cooperative organization of labor unions in California) had as its objective the pooling of "the collective bargaining power of 1.75 million workers in the state of California, to ensure the greatest return for our health dollar, to secure an effective voice for the consumer for providing and planning health, and to establish the machinery for monitoring the cost and quality of health care services and preventing abuse."[1]

The Poor as Consumers

"Consumer" and "community" sometimes have come to mean the poor and disadvantaged, excluding other groups. Until recently, the poor, and especially the disadvantaged minority groups, had little chance to say or do anything that directly affected their health care. An affluent individual who was dissatisfied with his health care could find alternative sources. He could change doctors or insist on going to another hospital. But the poor patient had no such effective economic "vote." If he did not like the clinic, his only alternative was to stay away. So it is not surprising that the consumer movement has concentrated on gaining power for—or at least input from—those who up to now have had neither.

This emphasis on the poor consumer often to the exclusion of other groups has been unfortunate. Disregard for groups which represent the traditional power base has elicited tensions in consumer-provider relations. A group of consumers who apparently are dissatisfied with their health care and are often neglected today are not poor at all, but middle class: small businessmen, residents of rural areas, professionals and white-collar workers, and others whose right to health care is limited by geography, manpower shortages, lack of resources, and finances, and who have had neither the clout of the labor unions nor the power of the medicare and medicaid programs to fight their battles for them.

This is regrettable, because everyone who is a consumer should have some degree of representation. A hospital that serves a multifaceted patient population should avoid paying inordinate attention to any one group at the expense of others. At the same time, the hospital must pay attention to its resource providers in order to have the wherewithal to take care of resource consumers.

Traditional hospital trustees are in fact consumers and consumer representatives. To be effective, they are going to have to see that institutions work cooperatively together in the interests of the consumer.

Involvement v. Satisfaction

Consumer involvement and consumer satisfaction are different. Satisfaction to the consumer is essential whether or not there is involvement. Some critics argue that involvement of consumers in decision making is necessary if good service is being rendered. Such arguments fail to consider whether the service being rendered is what the consumer really wants. A captive audience has no options.

There have been instances when the provider wanted to provide preventive and comprehensive services, but the consumer wanted only crisis intervention service. The poor whose most immediate concerns are food, shelter, jobs, and education may rank health as a low priority. These consumers may want an emergency room where they can be seen immediately. Providers have established well-baby clinics, and consumers have complained that they have nowhere to go when their babies are sick!

Such different perspectives demand that a provider consider the value of consumer involvement. A provider may be satisfying consumer demands and still not be providing what he really needs. In other words, does the professional know better than the consumer?

Rigid geographic, community-oriented organization of health care does not necessarily satisfy consumers. If an individual residing near a community mental health care center is dissatisfied with his treatment approach, he has only one choice — stay away and receive no care.

Consumer involvement in community mental health center programs has not guaranteed their quality or their ability to meet the needs or desires of the consumers. Individuals who do not want to receive care in their own neighborhoods, who may want to go elsewhere, are locked in. What kind of voice do they have? Yet they are consumers, too. Geographic organization and consumer involvement do not necessarily mean a perfect, or even a better, solution.

One of the dilemmas of hospital management today is that promises made by the political sector have exceeded the resources available to meet those promises. Ambulatory care, for example, is one of the current panaceas. But ambulatory care without adequate financing, organization, and manpower will not work any better than other elements of the health care system.

A great deal of the criticism of health services today has come from politicians' creating expectations without providing the means for satisfying those expectations. Rather than admit that the government promised what it is not going to deliver, politicians search for villains, and the easiest targets are the hospital, the administrator, and the medical profession.

Consumers rightfully may be asking for certain services. But the institutions may not have the means to deliver them, either in terms of manpower, or finances, or space, and the government is not helping to find these means.

The present Administration has promoted the development of the health maintenance organization to guarantee both cost efficiency and comprehensive quality care. However, there is considerable evidence to prove that cost efficiency may be gained at the expense of quality and people-oriented service — the kind of amenities people want. Without a specific and effective mechanism to protect the consumer, production-line techniques, long waiting periods, and excessively tight utilization criteria may become commonplace features of the future ambulatory health base, especially if programs are underfunded.

Role of the Administrator

Who is in fact concerned with the patient? The administrator is the institutional person with the best chance of filling that role. The administrator is the only person in the hospital concerned with the total range of services, and therefore with meeting human needs. He has a vested interest in keeping the patient, the physician, and everyone else satisfied, if only because satisfied customers keep his institution financially viable.

The administrator is concerned with the welfare of the patient, the physician, the employes, and the community because, as a visible leader of a highly visible institution, he *has* to be concerned. He is the person upon whom all concerns and responsibilities converge. In spite of the diverse and conflicting pressures on him, only the administrator can make the system work — by synthesizing economic reality with demands from consumers and the desires of physicians.

The administrator knows that his responsiveness is the only way to minimize consumers' needs to express their concerns and dissatisfaction through governmental action or the courts, and that responsiveness is the best way to maximize the public's support for health programs as a priority.

Consumer-Provider Relationship

It is especially difficult for the administrator to be responsive to the needs of his consumer, the patient, because the consumer-provider relationship in a hospital is different from that in any other business or industry. Hospitals control neither the design and distribution of their product nor the demand for their services. They cannot even be assured that their product will be paid for once delivered. Between the hospital provider and the health care consumer stand layer upon layer of intermediaries—physicians, insurers, citizens' planning groups, and government agencies—that in fact control the choices, exercise the options, and make the decisions that are accomplished on more or less a one-to-one basis in virtually any other consumer-provider exchange.[2]

Today the administrator is a broker—the man in the middle. The administrative role offers unlimited responsibility with severely limited authority; the administrator seems to be all-powerful, all-controlling, but he acts from comparative weakness. However, by judicious use of his limited power, he *can* move the system.

The consumer movement has not yet come to terms with the responsiveness of the individual doctor, as opposed to that of the hospital. Consumers express problems about medical care or about doctors in the abstract, but they always emphasize the relationship between the individual and the institution.

When the patient goes to a physician in his private office, the doctor—the "target of expectation"—is the actual provider. But if he goes to the hospital's ambulatory care service, the doctor is still the primary provider, but the target of expectation is the institution. If the care is unsatisfactory, the hospital, not the doctor, is blamed.

The patient's demands on the institution are greater than his demands on his own physician. If his doctor is inconsiderate in the office, the patient often shrugs off such treatment as human nature. But if a doctor is inconsiderate in the hospital, the institution is to blame.

For the patient of the private physician, the hospital is an extension of his physician. He trusts his doctor; therefore, he trusts the hospital. On the other hand, for the patient being seen at the hospital clinic, the doctor is an extension of the hospital, i.e., the doctor is "good," because he practices at a "good" hospital, or the hospital is "bad" because the doctor leaves much to be desired.

The consumer's failure to recognize the differences between the physician and the hospital work many times to his disadvantage. Administrators know that many of the worst and yet justified complaints consumers have about hospitals are due to health professionals', including physicians', failure to respond to the need for change. Because hospitals cannot do without physicians, they sometimes accede to physician demands even when they doubt their validity.

Hospital-consumer relationships also are strained by government's attempt to police physicians through the hospital by means such as utilization review. For example, the patient who believes he is being sent home too soon blames the hospital, not his doctor.

The rationale for involving consumers in health services planning and evaluation has been accepted by not only the National Health Council but by the American Hospital Association, the California Hospital Association, and other spokesmen for the health care industry. Also, the rationale is written into legislation, e.g., the Partnership in Health Bill (PL 89-749).

In a major document entitled "Statement on Consumer Representation in Governance of Health Care Institutions," the AHA Board of Trustees declared that consumers should have a voice at the "policy making and program planning levels" in the nation's health care system.[3] A California Hospital Association policy statement called on its member hospitals to be "increasingly responsive to, and aware of, needs expressed by members of their communities, either as individuals or through appropriate groups."[4]

But consumer involvement has not been a notable success when attempted through community advisory groups and patient advocates, and no effective national organization of health consumers exists to tackle meaningfully the inadequacies that consumers perceive in the health care delivery system. An effective consumer group interested in health and hospitals, while it might make things uncomfortable for the status quo, might well be the voice that could have significant influence in legislative and administrative quarters. Such influence could prevent the government attacks on existing health care institutions. Hospitals probably have more to lose by resisting an intelligent, involved consumerism than by supporting it.

Before consumer involvement can be effective for the institution and meaningful to the consumer, some definitions must be established. The theory that individuals who use clinics should operate those clinics is a fallacy. Individuals who understand that they do not have the competence to be doctors or nurses nevertheless believe that they are capable of being institutional managers.

The roles in which consumers can make meaningful recommendations and participate in meaningful decisions must be separated from those in which they cannot. Three issues are involved:

1. policy, i.e., establishing goals and objectives;
2. resource allocation, i.e., examining the feasibility of those goals and objectives; and
3. style of implementing them.

The latter involves the facility's attitude toward and concern for the patient as a dignified human being.

For example, a hospital must decide if it is going to concentrate on additional inpatient services or shift to ambulatory care. Its decision to develop ambulatory services that are valid for the community is a matter of policy. Its recognition that all services cannot be provided for every member of the community is a matter of resource allocation. The hospital must decide what specific ambulatory services it is going to offer, and when it has made that decision, it must decide how these services will be provided, i.e., with human dignity, patient convenience, or assembly line production.

The consumers' needs are not ignored in these decisions, but the hospital must take into consideration what resources are available in terms of dollars, politics, and people. The consumers may want a service which the hospital is unable to provide because its skills are limited.

However, the consumer can help the hospital acquire the needed skill. A knowledgeable consumer can be a powerful force in helping hospitals get these resources allocated or funded by government.

Decision-making processes in the health field are necessarily complex, but complexity has been overlooked in most discussions of consumerism. Should hospitals make decisions on the basis of statistical studies of the needs of their community? Should they call all their clinic patients together and ask them?

User input—more than has been allowed before—is necessary. But more informed input—the kind that tackles the technical and professional issues which the technicians and professionals can answer—is also needed. Furthermore, the consumers involved in this process must be rational, sophisticated, and educated to the issues, at least on a broad scale.

The process can do without and cannot afford consumers who use rhetoric instead of reason and who have become professional fighters for issues unrelated to the system as it exists at present or as it needs to develop in the future. Consumers who use the health field for political reasons or to struggle for a power base are unwelcome and dangerous.

Team Approach

Consumer involvement need not be an adversary situation. The ultimate goal of the consumer and the provider is much the same: quality care to all in a way and at a cost that can be afforded. A team approach can be taken, provided the consumers are not trying to take over management and the institution does not totally ignore the users.

The priorities of the institution are not always those of the consumer. Hospitals must not ignore consumer priorities because they appear shortsighted and uninformed. If a hospital works with consumers on issues they care about, the consumers will eventually understand and help the hospital deal with its broader problems.

Administrators must not rely on "prefabricated models"—lists printed by government agencies that outline membership and purposes of advisory committees. Rather, consumer involvement, who the consumer spokesmen are and how they relate to the administration, should be tailored for each situation, based on the needs and objectives of the institution, its different communities, and their specific problems.

Hospital boards of directors always have been made up of influential individuals. Formerly, influence meant prestigious family, money, and the ability to underwrite a building. Today boards of directors still must be influential, but the type of influence has changed. Labor leaders, politicians, and consumers who can deliver large groups of voters are now needed. But if hospitals exchange a semieffective group of establishment people for an ineffective group of community people, they have much to lose and little to gain.

A banker is no less a consumer or a consumer representative than the next person. The important concern is to what extent he is sympathetic to, and to what extent he reflects, people's attitudes and needs. Any board of directors must be capable of delivering what the institution needs to meet the demands that are placed upon it. Consumer groups are influential not only if they tell the institution what it should be doing, but if they help the institution present its case in the arena where resources are allocated. In this sense, a community-based board is no different from an establishment-based board. The question remains: Can the board deliver?

Formerly, a board delivered money. Now it must deliver political clout and legislation. Boards may change in composition, but their basic function will remain the same.

The question central to consumerism is: How do institutions get governance that is responsive to the needs of people, and how do they get that input translated into action? If health care institutions develop effective consumer input mechanisms, these mechanisms will help give the health care delivery system the political clout and the number of supporters it needs to be able to deliver the product that consumers really want.

Rather than fighting change, and being afraid of it, hospitals should welcome individuals who can not only convey what they want and need, but can help get the resources to provide it. Only those who operate the institution can properly provide for its resources.

Summary

It is always easier to do things for or to people than to do things with people. Hospitals should strive to reduce the alienation of individuals from the institutions and staffs that claim to serve them and to provide these individuals with an opportunity to influence decisions that affect them.

Hospitals should provide for broad-based community or consumer participation in policy making, program planning, and resource acquisition, and progress toward those goals should be monitored via a similarly broad-based mechanism. However, operational responsibility must be delegated to management, and management must continue to be judged by its performance. There is no standard format or magic formula for consumer input. Advisory boards, regular board membership, standing committees, or ad hoc problem-oriented task forces are less important than consumer input work. While there are moral arguments in a democratic society for representation, good business practice is also important. Hospitals ignore both at their peril.

NOTES

1. Einar O. Mohn, "The Challenge . . . How Does the Voluntary System Respond?" *Hospital Forum,* January, 1969, pp. 8–24.

2. Lee F. Block and M. Elliot Taylor, "Bridging the Public Relations Gap Between Hospital Provider and Consumer," *Public Relations Journal,* August, 1972, p. 16.

3. American Hospital Association, "Statement on Consumer Representation in Governance of Health Care Institutions," Nov. 17, 1972.

4. California Hospital Association, "Policy Statement on Hospital-Consumer Relationships," July 14, 1971.

9. Introducing Marketing as a Planning and Management Tool

STEPHEN L. TUCKER

Reprinted from *Hospital & Health Services Administration* by Stephen L. Tucker by permission of the American College of Hospital Administrators, Winter 1977.

Marketing concepts have not provided significant input as tools for administrators of health care facilities in the voluntary sector. It has been suggested that the use of this standard management tool of the business sector by health administrators has been viewed as inappropriate, and that this viewpoint has caused health managers to neglect an important means to the furtherance of the goals of their organizations.[1]

Today, most hospital administrators would acknowledge that the well-being of their organization depends upon the attraction of resources to enable a hospital to meet the historical goals of patient care, teaching, and research. Attraction of the necessary resources and acceptance on the part of various publics of the hospital that the organization has attained its goals are vital to the long-term survival of the institution. Marketing, with its explicit concern for resource allocation and public acceptance, can provide useful tools for hospital managers working for the survival of the voluntary hospital.

An expanded concept of marketing, suggesting a broader application of the field and its techniques beyond the entrepreneurial sector, has been provided by Kotler in *Marketing for Non-Profit Organizations*: ". . . marketing is the analysis, planning, implementation, and control of carefully formulated programs designed to bring about voluntary exchanges of values with target markets for the purpose of achieving organizational objectives."[2]

Today's hospital environment has several characteristics that require new thinking and new approaches on the part of institutional managers. These characteristics include a leveled-off inpatient census for a significant number of hospitals,[3] as well as increasing scrutiny by regulating agencies, demand for new services, and demand for participation by a number of "publics" of the hospital.[4] As an adjunct to the processes of goal definition, evaluation of the achievements of the organization, and the development of institutional planning as an integral part of health administration activities, marketing can provide several useful concepts. It behooves the hospital administrator to take advantage of those aspects of the marketing discipline that will provide assistance in meeting the changing demands placed upon the organization and its management group.

The concept of hospital "publics" has been well identified by the practitioners of public relations in the hospital environment.[5] At the same time, the multiplicity of forces (or publics) that impinge upon the hospital in its planning activities and its day-to-day operations is widely recognized.[6] Marketing, particularly the notion of exchange relationships, integrates the concepts of the identification of the "publics" of the hospital, the influential forces operating upon the organization, and the growing organization efforts seen in institutional planning. Many relevant exchange relationships exist for the hospital. Two of these relationships are exchanges with patients and exchanges with the medical staff.

Exchanges with Patients

Patients desire those aspects of care identified as "amenities" by those involved in the delivery of health care. A hospital desires, in its part of the exchange, to be the patients' hospital-of-choice. The patients' desires might be dubbed as the "Holiday Inn syndrome." This desire of patients is both predictable and defensible. The performance of the hospital's housekeeping, maintenance, and dietary departments; and the attitudes of hospital personnel vis-à-vis the patient as a guest and not as an inanimate object of medical care delivery, are elements of patient satisfaction. This examination of "exchange systems" does not neglect the patient's stake in the technical-professional aspects of the hospitalization. However, these technical-professional aspects are, for the most part, placed in the hands of the admitting physician, third-party payors, governments, and other parties representing the patient's interest.

Amenities or New Equipment

If the hospital is to meet the expectations of the patient and thereby be the patient's hospital-of-choice, it is a legitimate management priority to provide facilities and services that meet the patient's need for the amenities of care. As a result of this emphasis, persuasive arguments can be made for the necessity of expending scarce capital resources on patient accommodations within the physical plant. This has been a particularly difficult task for the manager because of the strong arguments for the expenditure of capital funds on technological equipment to deliver direct technical medical care in the institution that has little or no effect on the hospital's appearance or the patient's reaction to the hotel aspects of the hospital stay.

Hospital administrators may argue that there are limited areas in which a comparison between the hospital and the hotel is valid. But they should recognize that in the hospital's exchange relationship with the patient, the patient will start with that comparison. The hospital and hotel industries differ substantially in the emphasis each places on meeting client expectations regarding several of these "hotel aspects." For example, hospitals take great pride in offering selective menus. Compared with the hotel industry, this is not an exceptional accomplishment. It is, rather, an achievement that should have been realized before it was. Furthermore, a choice between two entrees which must typically be made 24 to 36 hours prior to eating the meal, is not, from the patient's viewpoint, a remarkable achievement. Selective menus are not, in the typical hospital, an amenity at the "Holiday Inn" level. The hospital is falling short of providing its proper part of the exchange. The administrator's rejoinder, that total food costs are being brought in at a per-day cost that is less than the typical cost of the single restaurant dinner, is not known by, nor would it be particularly persuasive to, the patient who is aware that the total hospital bill far exceeds $100 per day.

Again, viewing the patient's need in the context of an exchange between the patient in the hospital, strong justification can be found for expenditures in employee educational and training programs that emphasize the role of all employees in meeting patients' needs. The emphasis of the hotel industry on this aspect of their provision of service stands in sharp contrast to the hospital's efforts in these areas. The total exposure of a patient to hospital personnel far exceeds the exposure of the patient to the admitting physician. A patient may be expected to respond to the inquiry, "Who did you see most during your hospital stay?" with the answer: "The nurse's aide on the day shift," not "My doctor." The total impression of that patient concerning his or her stay is heavily influenced by the interaction between the patient and that nursing aide. How much of the aide's training was spent on recognizing and coping with the socio-emotional needs of the patient as opposed to the physical tasks of the nurse's aide's job?

Exchanges with the Medical Staff

The admitting physician desires services in the hospital which facilitate patient care. In the exchange with the medical staff, the hospital desires to be the physician's hospital-of-choice for the admission of patients. Recognizing this exchange relationship, hospital management can provide services and an approach to relationships between the institution and its medical staff which will assist in reaching the hospital's goals.

The technical resources demanded by a high quality medical staff create heavy and continuing demands on the hospital organization for both capital expenditures and skilled personnel. The rate of technological change in medical equipment and the concomitant centralization of technically dependent care in the hospital is widely acknowledged.[7] The physician is expected to demand the full panoply of specialized resources that are appropriate to the hospital's size, geographic location, and service specialization. The first of such resources the hospital management must provide is the technological hardware necessary to meet current medical care standards. This demands a recognition that continual capital investment is necessary for the operation of the hospital. Where these demands for hardware are legitimate in terms of congruence with the goals and abilities of the institution, management's recognition of the necessity of capital expenditure is a part of the dynamic exchange between hospital organization and the medical staff. This recognition may assist in justifying the generation of capital on a continuous basis through any of the appropriate mechanisms of operating surpluses, the assumption of debt, the use of unearned income, and the use of the relatively small portion of needed cash which is obtained through depreciation. With both management and corporate boards aware of the small proportion of funds available through unearned income and the difficulty encountered by a number of hospitals in generating operating surpluses, there is increasing reliance upon the assumption of debt as a means of raising capital.[8] Many hospital management groups and governing bodies may be discomforted by the necessity of assuming debt, but the continuous rejuvenation of the organization's technical capabilities is a necessary part of the exchange relationship between the hospital and its medical staff. This reasoning offers a useful addition to the more obvious justifications, such as the fact of growing technological dependence for the delivery of medical care, continual technical obsolescence of a significant amount of diagnostic and treatment equipment, and the need to match the technical capabilities of competitors.

Hospital administrators know that their individual organizations cannot meet all of the demands for hardware that will be generated by a dynamic medical staff. With the advent of third-party review of decisions that were previously made entirely within the organization, both the process of formal preparation for review (requiring the explicit delineation of a number of factors that are critical in the decision-making process that may not have been specifically addressed without the impetus of the external review process) and the outside review itself (with the possibility of a rejection of a proposed project by a force external to the organization) might be helpful to the exchange relationship from the point of view of hospital administrators. With extensive documentation required by the third parties, and a proportion of the demands for capital expenditures being withdrawn internally as a result of such documentation, and with the above-mentioned possibility of rejection of the proposal by the third party, it may be more difficult for the medical staff to view the rejection of a capital expenditure request purely as a failure of management to fulfill its expected part of the exchange relationship. With the influence of outside forces more clearly in focus, negative responses to medical staff capital demands may not be so readily viewed as unilateral management failures.

Medical Staff Conveniences

At a more personal level, the medical staff needs can be seen as a desire for convenience in delivering the physician's professional services to the patient. Convenience depends to some extent upon the physical plan of the institution, with such elements as its communications systems, parking lots and physicians' entrances. Despite the built-in limitations of the physical plan, the hospital administrator should strive to insure that these aspects of the medical staff members' desires are attended to in realistic fashion. These desires can be considered "hygiene factors" as proposed by Herzberg.[9] Even equipped with a theoretical explanation for the impact of these factors, it is easy to underestimate the need for the paging system to operate, for consultation requests to be promptly delivered, and for the parking lot gates to work correctly. There is evidence that hospital administrators view this as a discouraging part of their total responsibility.[10] But from a viewpoint of the exchange relationship, these needs have significant importance to the institution.

A second of the more personal aspects of the exchange relationships between the medical staff member and the institution concerns freedom in terms of the individual professional practice. This desire appears to run contrary to the forces operating on the hospital and the physician. The hospital administrator needs no reminder of the threat of the PSRO activity as perceived by the medical staff member. In this arena it is difficult for the institution to provide for the physician's needs. But it might be helpful for the administrator to point out that the hospital also feels the pressures of increased outside review of medical practice and that these pressures are not due solely to the efforts of the institution's management. Third-party payors, including both the government and the Blues, lead the fray. It is not reasonable for the medical staff member to view these pressures as entirely attributable to the institution's efforts working in a direction contrary to the physician's desires. Educational efforts on the part of the hospital, demonstrating the source and extent of the forces being brought to bear on the hospital as well as the individual practitioner, may bring about the realization that utilization pressures are coming from all sides, not just from within the institution.

In addition to the needs of the medical staff member as a professional practitioner, the admitting physician desires that the nontechnical or non-health needs of the patient be met by the institution. These needs have been addressed in relation to the exchange system between the hospital and the patient. If the hospital can meet these needs in the manner discussed, this aspect of the exchange between the hospital and the physician is adequately fulfilled. For example, the medical staff member does not expect to have to complain for the patient concerning food, housekeeping, maintenance, or personnel attitudes; the hospital owes satisfaction of these elements directly to the patient as part of the exchange between the hospital and the patient.

Viewing the relationship between patient and hospital and medical staff and hospital in terms of the exchanges between each of these publics and the institution, sidesteps the issue of which of the forces dominate in the choice of a particular hospital as the site for the delivery of medical care. By focusing upon the exchange relationship, it can be seen that both the patient and the medical staff member have particular objectives to fulfill in exchange for their use of the hospital, and it is the task of management to meet these if the hospital is to be the institution of choice.

The use of marketing concepts focusing on the relationship between the institution and its various publics as a series of exchanges provides a useful addition to the traditional tools of the hospital manager. By examining the desires of the patient and the medical staff and assessing the ability and effectiveness of the institution in satisfying these desires, the hospital manager is more completely equipped to promote the institution as the hospital-of-choice. This approach can be used effectively in relation to a list of publics beyond patients and the medical staff. A representative list of publics within the institution starts with employees, where union contract negotiations can be seen as a manifestation of the concepts of the demand for specific exchanges between the organization and an important public. Additional publics internal to the hospital include the corporate board, volunteers, and donors.

External to the hospital, groups with whom today's hospital must establish an equilibrium of exchanges include government at municipal, state, and federal levels, planning agencies, accrediting groups, other health facilities, third-party payors, consumer groups, and the media. Members of the institutional management responsible for dealing with each of these groups should find it useful to look at the institution's reciprocal relationships or exchanges with each of the groups to arrive at a more complete understanding of the needs of each party and a maximization of the benefits of the relationship.

NOTES

1. Charles M. Ewell, "Practical Plagiarism for Health Services Administration," *American Journal of Public Health* 64 (March, 1974): 233–37.

2. Philip Kotler, *Marketing for Non-Profit Organizations* (Englewood Cliffs, New Jersey: Prentice-Hall, Inc., 1975), p. 5.

3. Paul Ebers, "Hospital Indicators," *Hospitals* 48 (16 November 1974): 21.

4. Everett A. Johnson, "Goodbye, Tight Little Island," *Administrative Briefs* 9 (April, 1975): 1–5.

5. American Society for Hospital Public Relations, *A Basic Guide to Hospital Public Relations* (Chicago: American Hospital Association, 1973), p. 3.

6. John H. Knowles, "The Hospital," *Scientific American* 299 (September, 1973): 125–37.

7. Anne R. Somers, *Health Care in Transition: Directions for the Future* (Chicago: Hospital Research and Educational Trust, 1971), pp. 27–36.

8. Hospital Association of New York State, *Fourth Annual Voluntary Hospital Fiscal Pressures Survey* (Albany, New York: Hospital Association of New York State, October, 1975), and David E. Marine and John A. Henderson, "Trends in the Financing of Hospital Construction." *Hospitals* 48 (1 July 1974): 56.

9. Frederick Herzberg, Bernard Mausner, and Barbara B. Snyderman, *The Motivation To Work* (New York: John Wiley and Sons, 1959).

10. Samuel Davis and Stanley Henshaw, *Decision Analysis in Hospital Administration* (Washington, D.C.: Association of University Programs in Health Administration, 1974), pp. 7, 8.

10. This Hospital Holds Itself Accountable to Community

ANTHONY CONSTANTINE AND JAMES E. CASSIDY

Reprinted from *Modern Hospital* by James E. Cassidy and Anthony Constantine by permission of Crain Communications. © August 1969.

In a speech before the 1968 annual meeting of the American Hospital Association, Whitney Young, chairman of the National Urban League, noted that several hospitals had made "valuable beginnings" in their relationships with ghetto communities. Later, Mr. Young cited Metropolitan Hospital Center, New York, as one of the hospitals which qualified for that description.

No one at Metropolitan claims we have made more than some valuable beginnings. But we believe these initial tentative steps are forming a solid base from which we can reach our ultimate goal of bringing to the poor a quality of care that is at least equal to that provided by the best voluntary hospitals in the city.

Our efforts have been aided by the infusion of fresh administrative blood: seven key administrative positions have been filled within the last year. These new professionals are dedicated to the development of Metropolitan into one of the best hospitals in the city, not just the best city hospital.

One of the most important techniques of determining community needs is the face-to-face meeting. Administrators now attend meetings, within the community, at which all the problems that form the pattern of poverty—from drug addiction to housing, from sanitation to police protection—are discussed. This contact provides top administrators with the opportunity to meet community leaders and at the same time acquaint themselves with the conditions that affect all aspects of the community's existence.

Possibly because of these contacts, administrators have gone beyond their regular duties at times of special need in the community. One evening in December, for instance, the associate administrator for nursing services received a complaint from a local resident about the lack of heat or hot water for three days in buildings acquired by the city and scheduled to make way for a hospital expansion. The associate administrator personally visited the buildings to verify the complaint and then, at midnight, called the hospital administrator who in turn phoned the commissioner of hospitals who called the commissioner of real estate. Early the next day an inspector was in the building and by afternoon the heating system was working again.

Groups with special problems are invited to discuss their needs with the administrator and the hospital staff. Emphasis is placed on exchanging names so that important hospital personnel become accountable individuals in the eyes of community residents.

An example of this type of procedure was the change we made to accommodate a group of mothers who complained of difficulties in scheduling Head Start physicals for their children. Only a few lab tests were accomplished on their first visit, the mothers objected, and the complete physical took as many as four visits. Following a meeting between the mothers and representatives of hospital administration, pediatrics and the laboratories, it was decided that the procedure could be simplified by modifying certain lab schedules and slightly altering the examination.

The mothers were given the phone numbers of several administrators and told to call the administrator-on-duty at any time, day or night, if they had difficulties in the clinic or emergency room. This offer has been acted upon and the problems which instigated the telephone calls have been quickly solved in every case.

Metropolitan Hospital serves an area covering the midsection of Manhattan, from 42nd Street to 116th Street and from the Hudson River to the East River. The hospital has been served by a Community Advisory Board which was made up of professional people from the more affluent sections of this area. To give a voice in hospital affairs to those people who most use the hospital, three representatives from East Harlem were added to the advisory board. But, we realized, this would only be a stop-gap measure until representatives of the actual patient population could be included on the panel.

To gain the specific information needed to select a truly representative board, a detailed survey was undertaken by an independent organization. Using 20 per cent of the patient records as a sample, the surveyers determined that almost 60 per cent of the hospital's patients came from the east side above 92nd Street and another 24 per cent came from a parallel area on the west side. An ethnic and religious breakdown also was made.

Our present Community Advisory Board has appointed a nominating committee to search out new members who will be truly representative of the hospital's consumers. Eventually, the board will include representation from each major consumer group in the community.

Metropolitan also has attempted to make its outpatient department more responsive to the community. Although its OPD was one of the largest in the world, Metropolitan's outpatient services suffered from inadequate procedures and an obsolete philosophy. The services were unnecessarily fractioned and partitioned, often inflexible, and significantly impersonal. Resources and facilities were not adequately used.

A change in philosophy was the first requisite of an improved OPD. The staff was reoriented to view the patient as a part of his total environment rather than as a disease entity. The patient's sociological and socio-cultural background and the significance of his family dynamics were emphasized in the new approach.

An important and tangible aspect of this new philosophy is the conference nurse. In the obstetrics clinic, as an example, a conference nurse meets with the patient on her first visit and discusses everything from the patient's emotions concerning the pregnancy to the diet her condition requires. The patient is told about the services she may receive from the hospital's social service department and other departments. A diet is developed based on the patient's customary eating patterns and a special effort is made to substitute ethnic dishes for the foods in a prepared list.

Most important, a personal relationship is established between the nurse and patient at this initial conference. The patient then has someone to whom she can confide her problems during the pregnancy. The expectant mother is urged to call any time she has a question or to visit the nurse whenever she feels the need for a detailed discussion.

After a thorough examination by a doctor, the patient again meets with the conference nurse. The doctor's findings are explained and questions that the patient might be embarrassed to ask a doctor are answered. The patients are invited to attend a series of seven two-hour mothers' classes where they are prepared for delivery and the early care of their babies. These classes are conducted in both English and Spanish.

On each subsequent visit to the clinic, the patient meets with her conference nurse after the doctor's examination. All hospital admission forms are prepared in advance of confinement and the expectant mother is made completely familiar with the admissions process.

The conference nurse relationship is carried right through the hospital stay. The new mother is visited on the ward by her nurse, who helps with any questions or problems. Because the relationship is so long and firmly established, nurses find that patients speak much more freely with them than they would with a ward nurse.

The conference nurse concept is used in many other clinics as well.

Many East Harlem children leave for camp during the summer months. The physical exams these children require before embarking might have caused an administrative nightmare if the regular procedure of registration and appointment had been followed. When one of the local Boys Club leaders explained the difficulties to Metropolitan's administrator, special arrangements were made so that many of the regular formalities could be dispensed with in these examinations. In addition, extra staff was brought in so that the 1,000 physicals could be accomplished with relative ease.

To build interest in hospital and health care careers, local school groups have been invited to visit the hospital and receive in-depth orientation in various specialized areas. An open house recently was held for all members of the community. Several thousand people toured the hospital, received information on health care and careers, and informally chatted with administrators and other personnel. In this activity, as in all others, the hospital makes every effort to provide interpreters and to place bilingual employes where they will be best able to help non-English speaking patients and visitors.

Mothers of large families in the East Harlem area frequently were experiencing difficulty placing their children with friends or relatives while they brought an ill child to our OPD. To alleviate this problem somewhat, we extended pediatric clinic hours to 8 p.m. and now keep the clinic open on Saturday and Sunday from 2 p.m. to 6 p.m.

Community cooperation also has been sought in determining the disposition of the hospital's resources. For example, the community is being consulted on the utilization of a new 250 bed Community Mental Health Center. Plans are being made to hire and train as many neighborhood people as possible to staff the center.

A planning committee that considers long-range construction needs includes community representatives as well as administrators and physicians. The specific needs of the area are discussed and the recommendations agreed upon by the committee are presented to the community at large.

Members of the community participated in the planning for a $4.2 million crash program designed to improve present facilities. These renovations, which are currently underway, will result in an expanded outpatient department and emergency services wing. This program also will include improvements in our laboratories and radiology, which should help alleviate one of the most persistent community complaints: long waits for x-rays and lab tests.

Community reaction indicated a need for more family planning facilities and the desirability of improving the hospital's sensitivity to community needs. Accordingly, we now are considering a satellite family planning center and we are planning to add to our staff a full-time community-based hospital representative who will serve as liaison between the hospital and those it serves.

Each of these programs or steps has been a significant "beginning," but the most important accomplishment of the last year is intangible. That is the feeling of confidence and trust that is starting to characterize the relationships between the community and the hospital. This attitude manifests itself in a thousand little ways, but it is most apparent in comparisons with the community's former attitudes, which ranged from disapproval to outright condemnation.

11. Vox Populi—or Hearing the Voices of Your Public

SHIRLEY BONNEM

Based on two previously published articles, "Role of Public Relations in Marketing for Non-Profit Organizations," by Shirley Bonnem, in *Channels*, a newsletter of the Public Relations Society of America, December 1978; and "Good Marketing Helps a Hospital Grow," by Shirley Bonnem and Warren C. Falberg, in *Hospitals, Journal of the American Hospital Association*, June 1, 1977.

The ingredients needed to make a hospital successful are not easy to define. For some hospitals, however, the key to a successful institution may rest with an effective marketing program. Today a hospital does not ensure itself of success by simply being available to the public.

Simply stated, marketing involves exchange; it offers value in exchange for value.

The tools of marketing are analyses that reveal possible market segments and the ability of an organization to concentrate on those segments that have the greatest need and the largest volume. In applying marketing analysis to hospitals, administrators must address the following questions: What market need is the organization attempting to satisfy? How can the hospital's product be shaped to meet the needs of the intended market? Finally, how can the hospital communicate its intentions and deliver a product to individuals or groups at a cost that these people perceive to be reasonable?

The problems faced by the health care field, particularly hospitals, include issues of major restraints and a finite availability of resources. In addition, today's consumers of service are able, more than ever before, to choose among providers of service and to establish support and loyalty to the provider that gives the greatest satisfaction.

In response to these realities, the marketing approach to hospitals involves a perspective in which the management of resources must be dedicated to the purpose of serving and/or influencing an identifiable group of people in such a manner that both sides perceive exchanged values as the ultimate outcome. Rather than being all things to all men, hospital marketing involves the selection of target areas, or "publics." Accordingly, the long-term success of any marketing program must be judged by the amount of satisfaction that its programs and services generate among its identifiable publics.

Once the marketing program is understood, it can be applied to any institution. Often, the biggest obstacle in getting a program underway is resistance to the word marketing. Forget semantic distinctions; if necessary, do the work under any name.

Assuming that everyone from the board to the professional staff has endorsed the marketing program, don't proceed until there is a budget to do the work.

A marketing program should be directed to two major and several ancillary publics, namely, physicians, patients, the general populace within the Hospital's catchment area, nurses and volunteers. Only the first three publics are addressed here.

The Physician Public

Physicians are the "deciders," the people who select what they think they need for good patient care, where they want to perform the service and how they would like the support services to be organized.

One rarely finds a patient who resists a doctor when he or she refers that patient to a specific hospital.

A part of the physician marketing effort involves the determination of the needs of referring physicians and of the hospital's own medical staff. To accomplish this, one children's hospital designed and mailed a questionnaire to 3,900 physicians in the tri-state area of Pennsylvania, Delaware, and New Jersey. The questionnaire brought a 19 percent response and elicited major areas of praise and criticism. The hospital's marketing effort sought to capitalize on the areas of response that were praiseworthy and to find solutions to areas of criticism.

The area of the hospital receiving the most praise from physicians was the infant intensive care unit. This hospital built on the physicians' positive attitude toward the infant intensive care unit by opening an intermediate level of intensive care for older children. This 25-bed unit was a direct response to the expressed needs of a sizable group of physicians.

The hospital also sought to find solutions to the two major areas of criticism noted in the questionnaire—lack of ongoing communication with the referring physician and a need for more continuing education programs for physicians. To deal with these criticisms, the hospital asked for the cooperation of the physicians' community relations committee. This committee and the hospital's public relations department attempted to solve both problems.

In response to the need for improved communication, the hospital sent an open letter to all referring physicians outlining steps to be taken by the hospital to keep referring physicians aware of their patients' conditions. This program was implemented by the physicians' committee on community relations.

In light of the need for more continuing education programs, a schedule of lectures and seminars was sent to all physicians reached by the questionnaire. The hospital sent a brochure listing all meetings, seminars, and conferences for physicians to be held at the hospital. In addition, the hospital medical staff encouraged referring physicians to attend grand rounds and departmental conferences.

Although the hospital did not systematically determine whether or not physicians have noticed these changes, an increase of 2,000 patient days during the year following the survey seemed to be a positive indication.

The Patient Public

Knowing the patient's needs and meeting them reinforces a hospital's marketing efforts.

A one-person public relations department in a New England hospital persuaded the administrator that a miniature marketing audit was a good idea. First, a questionnaire was designed to see how the hospital was perceived by patients. The next step was to conduct the survey among a limited audience—"just to see how it went and to determine its effectiveness." The number of people who responded was astonishing. The expansion of the project should give the organization an accurate picture of itself.

There are four advantages to the approach. The first is to ease oneself into a relatively new discipline, and by doing so prevent the hospital administration and medical staff from feeling overwhelmed by "marketing." Two additional benefits: The public relations director was able to demonstrate the need for a self-audit by showing a concentrated response from a small group. Also the hospital family was offered an opportunity to see the usefulness of the program without feeling obligated to take on a huge effort without knowing what was involved.

In another example, a children's hospital learned from a survey of the patients' parents that although they appreciated having overnight facilities available to them, they felt "raunchy," "dirty," "messy," or "cruddy" the next day. Reason? Lack of showering facilities.

The hospital designated the bathrooms near its residents' on-call rooms as shower rooms for parents before 9 a.m. Parents were provided with a packet containing a towel, washcloth and soap. The availability of the showers gave parents a feeling that the hospital was concerned about them.

An urban teaching hospital contemplated installing closed-circuit television and expensive tapes to provide health care education to its waiting public in the emergency department. Before investing time and money in the project, the public relations director enlisted the help of volunteers in an effort to survey the captive audience. Purpose was to see how that particular segment of the public would respond to the closed-circuit education.

Anticipating positive response to the idea of television presentations—after all, isn't the country in love with the "tube"—the surveyors were astonished to find that these patients wanted their education from nurses. They did not want to watch video cassettes; they were not interested in health care education meetings; they did not care to read publications emphasizing consumer health education. The patients felt comfortable in a one-to-one setting with a nurse who would not judge the questions as too simple. In response to the survey the hospital assigned a nurse clinician to the project. The closed-circuit project was abandoned.

The Public at Large

While one phase of the hospital's marketing effort should be directed toward physicians and another to the patients, the hospital should make a thorough effort with the public at large. Projects can be undertaken to make the community aware of the role of the hospital such as sponsoring special events by health-oriented community organizations.

A Long Island hospital learned that the public was starved for knowledge about sexuality, the middle years and aging. It provided a lecture series in a community high school which conducted a program at night for area residents.

So interesting were the sessions that some of them were covered by local media, reinforcing the hospital's position as an institution concerned not only with the sick, but with the community's well-being.

Summary

One marketing objective of a hospital should be to educate its target markets—physicians, patients and the community-at-large—about the services and facilities of the hospital. In many cases the marketing effort should seek to reinforce the hospital's particular position in the community as a health care provider.

Marketing has begun to permeate the nonprofit sector, particularly in the health care field. Those who have confused the function with selling, or who have avoided its use because they think it will create an artificial need for certain services, should reconsider their position, particularly in view of increasing public support for a more "business-like" nonprofit sector. As consumers become more aware of what they want from agencies, not-for-profit institutions inevitably will be forced to engage in marketing to provide the proper mix of product, place, price and promotion.

HEALTH CARE MARKETING C.A.P.S.: SPECIFIC AREAS FOR MARKETING'S CONTRIBUTION

OVERVIEW

This section is key to this book because it outlines and provides examples from the literature of four areas where a marketing approach and point of view can contribute.

The first two articles set the tone for the four articles that follow. The first, "Entry Strategies for Marketing in Ambulatory and Other Health Delivery Systems," describes the degree of difficulty marketing faces in entering each level of medical care. It also isolates points of view that differ on marketing in the business and in the health care sectors that are particularly important for marketers with little experience in health care who are considering entering this field. The second article, "Marketing Health Care Services: The Challenge of Primary Care," reviews the traditional concepts and marketing litany (price, place, promotion, and product) with respect to health care delivery and primary care in particular. It reviews some of the techniques that can be used to approach the health care market.

The next four sections describe the specific areas, referred to as C.A.P.S., in which marketing approaches, techniques, and philosophies can contribute.

In preparing this volume, it became obvious that if marketing as a discipline useful to health care delivery was to survive the threat of becoming a fad, recognition must be given to an appreciation for the real differences between "similar" areas of the business and health care sectors. In business, these traditionally are referred to as pricing, the place of or form of distributing the product or service, the promotion, and the product. From a health care marketing point of view, C.A.P.S. refer to:

C. Consideration: This goes beyond "price" or cost to the consumer to include something of value given up by the consumer in exchange for health care services.

A. Access or availability: This goes beyond the word "place" used by the goods marketer to encompass the health care consumer's real concern.

P. Promotion: As with the goods marketer, it means advertising and personal selling, but in health care marketing it emphasizes the roles of public relations and health education as well as introducing the roles of atmospherics and incentives.

S. Service Development: This simply points out the shift from the "products" of the goods marketer to the "services" of the health care marketer.

The danger for health care marketing lies in the temptation to transfer techniques directly from the business sector into the health care sector without appreciating the differences. This danger may be ameliorated by the use of health care marketing C.A.P.S. Each of these areas will be discussed in more detail in the introduction to each of those four sections.

12. Entry Strategies for Marketing in Ambulatory and Other Health Delivery Systems

PHILIP D. COOPER, RICHARD MAXWELL, AND
WILLIAM KEHOE

Reprinted, with permission, from *The Journal of Ambulatory Care Management*, Vol. 2, No. 2,
May 1979, by permission of Aspen Systems Corporation, © 1979.

The concept of marketing is relatively new to the health care industry and has only recently begun to receive attention as a viable management tool. However, marketing concepts and techniques have important applications to health care, including ambulatory care. In
order to appreciate these applications, it is essential to understand the
health care environment.

THE HEALTH CARE ENVIRONMENT

PSROs

During the 92nd session of Congress, 1971 to 1972, the Social Security Act was amended to create what have become known as PSROs for
the purpose of assessing the care provided to patients under Title V
(Maternal and Child Health and Crippled Children Services), Title
XIX (Medicare) and Title XX (Medicaid). PSROs are charged with
evaluating the necessity of services rendered by physicians to patients,
the appropriateness of the facilities where these services are rendered
and the quality of service or care provided.

HSAs

Several years later, the National Health Planning and Resource
Development Act established a process whereby local planning groups
called HSAs are to evaluate an area's health care services, manpower
and facilities. On the basis of this evaluation, the HSA is to develop
and implement a health care plan to meet identified needs and reduce
documented inefficiencies. In addition, the act calls for state CON laws
enabling HSAs to pass judgment on proposed capital expenditures by
hospitals, proposed increases or decreases in number of beds and proposed new services.

HSAs and PSROs are encouraged to interact and exchange data where confidentiality permits. Such information sharing can serve as a rational basis for allocation of health care resources. For example, where a region shows an above-normal number of inpatient days paralleled by a lack of ambulatory care facilities, nursing beds or other alternatives to hospitalization, a CON application for additional acute-care beds is likely to be denied in favor of care alternatives that do not require hospitalization. PSROs and HSAs thus have the potential to create a major shift in patient care patterns as well as affect the goods and services available for consumption.

Health Care Suppliers and Demanders

It is of interest to point out that individuals or institutions supplying health care services are not necessarily adhering to rational plans based upon accurate data from the surrounding area; they are more likely to be responding to immediate internal pressures. Adherence to rational area-wide plans is achieved either through voluntary cooperation or through negative reimbursement for services for which a CON has not been granted.

The physician plays an interesting role in the health care arena, establishing an agency relationship with the patient and thus becoming the actual demander of goods and services in the health care system. The PSRO acts to regulate that demand by determining what institution, services, length of stay, etc. are appropriate for the physician's patient. Likewise, the HSA mechanism serves to control or regulate the supply of institutions, facilities and services available to the physician as the demander. Consequently, the health care environment has become much more regulated, diminishing the prerogatives of management with regard to the expansion of services and facilities.

Technological Change

The advancement of medical technology and its application and delivery setting are also important in the health care environment. Twenty years ago, health care institutions could commonly be described as manpower intensive. Now it is more accurate to state that hospitals and ambulatory care facilities are intensive in terms of both manpower and capital. The most highly visible example of current technological development is the computerized axial tomography or CAT scanning recently introduced in the field of radiology. A CAT scanner, with a price of up to $750,000 for a single unit, is a diagnostic tool that provides the radiologist with a view of the body unavailable through conventional radiologic techniques. However, despite the remarkable advances in diagnostic capabilities made possible by CAT scanning, negative consumer attitudes have been created by the high cost of this technology to the individual patient. A typical charge for a CAT scan is $200 for the technician component, plus an additional $75 to $100 for the professional fee. This clash between the need for services and the cost of such services raises the thorny question of how much technology is enough. Where do we draw the line?

Emergence of Marketing

Health care professionals are experiencing major changes in attitudes toward techniques such as marketing and advertising. Increasingly, physicians are advertising services, as are ambulatory care facilities and hospitals; this trend is likely to be furthered by recent court rulings regarding lawyers and their freedom to advertise.

Perhaps the most difficult aspect of the marketing of services by health care institutions relates to consumer attitudes toward health care. During the Johnson administration, the belief that health care is everyone's right became popular, and it is now firmly engrained in much of society. Today's health care consumers demand that care be of high and consistent quality yet be provided to them at a low cost. The issue which must inevitably be faced is the need to ration our health care resources. This will almost certainly lead to a conflict between the perceived right to health care and the need to plan for the development and deployment of our resources.

ENTRY POINTS FOR MARKETING HEALTH CARE

Preventive Health Care

Marketing generally makes its most notable contributions in situations where supply is greater than demand. Thus its easiest and most logical point of entry into the health care field may be in the area of preventive health care services, which in most cases are ambulatory. A clear example of what it can do in this area is the recent intensified campaign by various professional societies in the United States to make people aware of the value of immunization, its availability through local health departments and its extremely low price—indeed often free.

Somewhat more difficult to promote are broad-based efforts to educate people to the long-term benefits of preventive health care measures, both to their health and their pocketbooks. For adults to seek preventive care for themselves is a voluntary act, as is the purchase of many products. Thus one would expect marketing techniques to be of value in encouraging preventive care behavior patterns. Unfortunately, existing behavior patterns on the part of many adults are strongly oriented toward curative medical care on an episodic basis. Thus the issues and factors become larger than simply marketing, requiring a number of things to happen.

The most interesting (yet at the same time distressing) factor is the reimbursement of providers by third party payers who cover the vast majority of people in the United States. In most cases, health insurance covers some portions of outpatient care associated with specific illnesses but generally does not provide reimbursement for routine ambulatory items such as a physical check-up. This leaves the burden of both seeking and paying for preventive care squarely on the shoulders of the consumer. A preventive care orientation is antithetical to the expectations and behavior patterns associated with third party health insurance.

The challenge in marketing preventive care is to prove to consumers that by purchasing this service they will decrease their health care expenditures in the long run. This may be extremely difficult when consumers are faced with the fact that they are purchasing health care coverage through their employers and do not have the option of taking those premiums in their paychecks. Additionally, the high cost of hospitalization virtually demands that people maintain third party coverage.

(For a more comprehensive overview of the opportunities for a marketing approach see **Marketing and Preventive Health Care.**[1])

Primary Care

Health care is generally divided into three levels: primary care, which is ambulatory and is defined as first contact, comprehensive care over a long period of time (with this definition one moves away from the concept of episodic medicine and toward that of continuity of care); secondary care, which can be defined as care received by patients after being referred from their primary physician to a specialist; and (at the highest and most sophisticated level) tertiary care, which is almost exclusively an inpatient form of care provided by highly specialized physicians using extremely sophisticated technology most often found in teaching hospitals.

The marketing of primary care services may seem a somewhat difficult entry point into the health care field, but may in fact prove more fruitful than marketing preventive care. Through a long-term relationship between patients and physicians in a primary care service (that is, family practice, general internal medicine and pediatrics), an understanding and confidence is developed that allows physicians to address not only illnesses but nondisease problems which may affect the patients' health. By virtue of patients' long-term relationship with physicians, they can receive information regarding how to improve their health in the long run as well as working to cure their immediate problems. Ongoing contact with primary care physicians facilitates activities such as patient education. Thus primary health care has many highly desirable and marketable aspects.

Secondary and Tertiary Care

Probably marketing's most difficult entry point would be through secondary- and tertiary-level health care services, where demand is almost universally a nonvoluntary act based on an acute need identified by a primary care physician. Secondary and tertiary care are almost always referral activities in which the service is demanded not by consumers but by the consumers' physicians acting as their agents. Where this is not true, demand for such care is usually related to a severe injury or illness necessitating immediate medical or surgical attention. Thus secondary and tertiary care do not appear at first glance to be promising areas for marketing.

However, research on potential markets can play an extremely useful role in the efforts of hospitals and HSAs to develop rational plans for a health service area—especially in regard to sophisticated, expensive services at secondary and tertiary levels. By assessing the marketplace and projecting potential needs and demands for these services, marketing can help distribute health care resources more effectively and rationally. Indeed, the greater requirement for more information brought about by the CON legislation makes it desirable for marketing studies to be undertaken prior to the investment of large amounts of capital in new buildings or equipment for hospitals and other delivery systems. Table 1 provides an overview of entry points discussed in the preceding sections.

Demarketing

Another application of marketing in the health care field may occur through what is known as "demarketing"—that is, a systematic mar-

Table 1 Marketing's Entry Points to Health Care: A Quadrivariate
Analysis

Entry Point	Perceived Attitude of Health Care Community Toward Marketing	Perceived Applicability of Marketing in the Health Care Area	Perceived Difficulty of Entry	Viable Entry Strategy
Preventive health care	Increasing acceptance	Very high	Little	Highly tactical (position marketing as a tool for advertising, research, etc.)
Primary care	Some acceptance	High to moderate	Some	Tactical with some strategic
Secondary care	Low acceptance	Moderate to low	Much	Increasingly strategic with some tactical
Tertiary care	Very low acceptance	Low	Extreme	Highly strategic (position marketing in a planning and policy focus mode)

keting effort aimed at **decreasing** consumption of a given item or
service. If national health insurance is enacted, demand for health care
may increase greatly. A recent study of the effects of a national health
insurance package providing full coverage on demand for all ambulatory care services estimates conservatively that such coverage would
increase 30 percent.[2] In such a situation, demarketing could play a
significant role. Just as the consumption of electrical power during
peak demand periods has been demarketed, it may also be possible to
demarket demand for physician services—either by educating consumers to be more discriminating about the instances when health
care is truly needed, or by convincing physicians that "physician ex-
tenders" (nurse practitioners or physician assistants) can appropri-
ately and effectively treat minor illnesses and thus allow the physician
to concentrate on more complex cases.

DIFFICULTIES IN APPLYING MARKETING TO HEALTH CARE

Marketing concepts are still very new to the health care field and are
not yet fully accepted by health care administrators as useful management tools directly applicable to health care. Also, their applications to health care have not yet been fully refined.

Definition and Measurement

Perhaps the most obvious problem centers around how one defines and measures success. Those who market products often measure success in terms of a few percentage points gained in their share of the market. But market-share assessment has extremely limited application in the health care field; here success needs to be viewed on a different scale. In the area of immunology and preventive medicine, for example, successful treatment is not measured by small increments of gains toward eradication of the illness; rather it is measured when 100 percent of the market has been reached. A pitfall for the person with a marketing background, new to the health care industry, is to be satisfied with small gains.

Meaning of Marketing

Another problem that immediately surfaces is the stigma of the word "marketing." To many in health care, marketing is equated with hard sell. It is incumbent upon marketing professionals to attempt to overcome such preconceptions and demonstrate to health care professionals the true value of marketing concepts and techniques. And those working in health care should be open to the ways in which marketing can contribute to their field.

Profit Orientation

The belief that health care delivery systems should not be profit oriented needs to be reexamined. Social mores hold that making money from the sick and the infirm is not acceptable; however, it must be recognized that these earnings represent the physicians' livelihood as well as the basis for financial solvency of the health care delivery system. The business of a clinic or hospital is to provide needed services to patients and to offer an economical setting for physicians to treat patients. In some cases this requires making available certain services that are guaranteed loss leaders, the emergency room being the classic example.

In order to offset these money-losing services, others must be operated at a profit. The value of marketing research in this setting is obvious. It can help the administrator prudently select services by assessing their profitability and then measuring it against patient needs. Despite this help, the ambulatory or hospital administrator is often faced with the conflicting goals of maintaining the financial integrity of the institution while providing services to people at time of great need with little regard for cost.

Consumer Orientation

In a free market system, the consumer is king. In the present health care system, with the physician acting as the patient's agent, there are obvious limits on consumer choice and the consumer's control over the care he or she receives. The physician in effect becomes a benevolent dictator for the patient. For example, most potent pharmaceuticals are unavailable without a physician's prescription, surgical services are unavailable unless a physician decides that an operation is necessary, admissions to a hospital do not occur unless a physician admits the patient, etc. It is important to recognize this phenomenon, for it establishes definite boundaries to the key marketing concept of consumer orientation.

Problems of this sort will demand patience and understanding of marketers working in health care and open minds on the part of health care administrators. Perhaps even more important is the need for physicians to become oriented toward those services whose development will allow the demarketing of traditional health care services. A stronger preventive care orientation among physicians requires a substantial change in medical school training and emphasis. Young physicians are a primary contact point with the public in general, and it is reasonable to assume that the public will assimilate their health care orientations to a great extent. In addition, it is necessary to bring about a change in the third party reimbursement system to include the costs of preventive care.

After reviewing the changes occurring in the health care environment and the move toward a preventive emphasis in health care, it seems that marketing and some of its basic concepts have the potential to be of benefit, particularly to those involved in health care administration. However, a marketer should realize that viewpoints and measures of success in health care may differ from those of business. On the other hand, managers of ambulatory and other medical care need to be receptive to methodologies and thought processes that go beyond the traditional ways of handling and evaluating the administration of medical care services. Perhaps the most difficult task is that of the marketing professional, who must clarify marketing concepts and values and then, with the help of health care administrators, implement those concepts within the health care delivery system in a meaningful and useful manner.

REFERENCES

1. Cooper, P. D., Kehoe, W. J. and Murphy, P., eds. *Marketing and Preventive Health Care: Interdisciplinary and Interorganizational Perspectives* (Chicago: American Marketing Association, 1978).

2. Newhouse, J. P., Phelps, C. E. and Schwartz, W. B., "Policy Options and the Impact of National Health Insurance." *New England Journal of Medicine* 296:24 (June 13, 1974) p. 1345–1359.

13. Marketing Health Care Services: The Challenge of Primary Care

ROBIN E. MACSTRAVIC

Reprinted from *Health Care Management Review*, Summer 1977, by permission of Aspen Systems Corporation © 1979.

The marketing of health services has not, up to now, been a major focus in the management of health care organizations. Partly, this reflects a popular misunderstanding of the nature and purpose of marketing itself. Another reason has been the fact that hospitals and most other organizations for the delivery of health care "sell" their services through physicians, rather than directly to the consumer. Despite popular misconceptions regarding what marketing is and does, this "alien" discipline should be of particular interest to managers of health care organizations in the future.

WHAT IS MARKETING?

The most common notion as to what marketing is tends to equate it with selling and advertising. The very word "marketing" may evoke overtones of hucksterism and manipulation of human behavior to sell people more than they really need. Such efforts would obviously be unsuitable, unethical or even illegal in health care. This limited view of marketing is inaccurate, however. Marketing covers the planning and management of all transactions between an organization and its constituents.

As pointed out by Kotler and others in the marketing field, the marketing of health services involves analyzing the current state of transactions with supporters, employees and regulators of organizations as well as its clients.[1] With a focus on patients, marketing includes identifying and evaluating current levels of utilization, and asking, for example:

- Are appropriate amounts of services being used, in terms of patient needs and the organization's capacity?
- Are the right types of services being used?
- Are services being used when most appropriate?

In addition to managing current utilization (e.g., so as to reduce nonemergency use of emergency room services, or to smooth out variations in demand for inpatient care), marketing can and does provide ways to program new services or increase use of existing programs.

Marketing encompasses the analysis and management of four factors essential to the delivery of health care:

Product: the type of service to be offered—preventive, diagnostic, therapeutic, etc., especially viewed in terms of the benefits the service provides to the patient—relief from pain or anxiety, longer life, less disability, etc.

Place: how the service will be delivered to the patient—the location, hours, referral mechanism, etc., which determine the extent and mode of access to the product.

Price: not only the charge made for the service (which often isn't paid directly by the patient anyway), but everything the organization requires the patient to go through in order to utilize the service.

Promotion: how and what the prospective patient learns about the organization and the services it offers—how the patient can become aware of services offered, develop an interest in using a service, decide to use it, actually utilize it, use it regularly, recommend the organization to friends, etc.

The analysis and management of these four factors may be geared to reducing the level of, smoothing out fluctuations in, changing the clients of, or increasing the utilization of existing services offered by the health care organization. They must also be considered in developing new or expanded services.

The concepts and techniques used in the field of marketing have been developed, employed and refined over decades of use in areas outside the health industry. While there are substantial differences between the application of marketing theory to health care organizations and prior applications of marketing, the purposes and functions are common. If there are ways in which the marketing discipline can be used effectively to manage existing health services or develop new and expanded ones, then both the organization and community benefit.

APPLICATION TO HEALTH CARE

There have been some recent attempts by those in the marketing field to describe the application of marketing logic to health care and other social services. Kotler has provided both a general discussion of marketing as an approach to social change,[2] and suggestions for some specific applications to the marketing of health services.[3] These suggestions have been reinforced by Zaltman and Vertinsky and most recently by Crane *et al.*[4,5] All these authors have offered useful conceptual models for application to health services. They have opened the way to greater understanding and acceptance of marketing principles in health services development.

Clearly, if marketing is understood as the facilitation of transactions between producer and consumer, it can easily be translated to apply to the facilitation of exchanges between health service provider and patient. The models suggested by Kotler and Crane both are based on identifying what health services the community needs and determining how best to deliver those services.[6,7] This has been the specific focus of health services planning and development for years. Unfortunately, the suggestions for marketing applications have been made in the marketing literature, and rarely if ever repeated in health literature.

Although there have been some specific applications of marketing principles in practice by the health system, by and large, these have been limited. A number of authors have described the marketing of family planning services as a successful application, though chiefly in terms of promotion.[8-13] In the past five years, a great deal of attention has been given the marketing of what was supposed to be the new wave of health services delivery: the health maintenance organization.[14] Specific suggestions have been made for adoption of marketing techniques in fund-raising, cancer detection and chest x-rays.[15,16,17] At least one author has called for marketing of hospital services.[18]

A number of recent developments have guided the more tradition-bound hospitals toward a newer application of marketing. Chief among these has been the growing dependence of hospitals on the cost-based reimbursement formulas of third party payers: the federal Medicare and Medicaid programs, Blue Cross health insurance, etc. As these third parties have increasingly cut back what they'll pay for, hospitals have had greater difficulty making up for bad debts and accumulating reserves through the dwindling numbers of private-paying patients. The prospect of a national health insurance program which would eliminate private patients entirely represents the ultimate crunch in this trend.

A second major factor has been the increasing pressure on hospitals to limit the amount of inpatient services it provides. Utilization review programs, PSROs and incentives for ambulatory care development are examples of specific pressures. The intended effect of these efforts, namely the minimization of inpatient utilization, requires "demarketing" of inpatient care and is a threat to the financial viability of hospitals. There are three obvious responses to this threat: increasing penetration into existing markets, increasing one's market so as to maintain inpatient utilization by serving a greater number of people, and developing other than inpatient services as a basis for increasing revenue. A hospital primary care program potentially combines all three responses.

PRIMARY CARE PROGRAMS

Hospitals have been moving into primary care for some time, though only gradually. Beth Israel Hospital in Boston reported on the conscious development of a primary care program in 1961.[19] More recently, the Robert Wood Johnson Foundation has authorized $30 million in grants to support up to 60 hospital-based primary care group practices.[20] A recent survey identified over 600 hospitals in various stages of development of primary care programs, including roughly 200 with programs in operation.[21]

These programs typically involve some portions of traditional marketing approaches. The *product* they offer is primary care with the added attraction of back-up capabilities of the hospital and continuity of care through common medical records.[22] The *price* is usually set at a level designed to be competitive with office-based physicians in contrast to the much higher fees prevailing for the care provided in emergency rooms.[23] For increasing numbers of hospitals, the *place* of contact between provider and consumer is adjusted by locating satellite centers in underserved areas, whether rural or urban.[24,25] The fourth factor in the marketing litany—the *promotion* of the centers— is common where hospitals have been reticent. This, too, however, is being addressed via such devices as news coverage on opening, the distribution of descriptive pamphlets, etc.

Primary care program development represents a substantially different challenge to the hospital in contrast to its traditional inpatient and emergency outpatient programs. Inpatients are brought into contact with the hospital through physician referrals. As long as sufficient numbers of doctors remain on the medical staff and continue admitting their patients, inpatient programs will succeed. In such a case, it is primarily the physician who must be maintained as a loyal client. For emergency services, hospitals have inherited the emergency and after-office-hours market from private physicians who wished to change their location and/or hours of practice.

The Market

The primary care market is comprised of potential patients who must be attracted directly rather than referred by physicians. Much of primary care (e.g., preventive or routine maintenance services) is perceived by most people as of marginal utility, and subject to personal choice as to whether and where to seek it. In contrast to inpatient or true emergency care, the patient is likely to have a definite notion as to what constitutes an acceptable quality of care, rather than rely on the expertise of the physician. In developing a primary care program, the hospital must attract patients directly, to make initial contact with and become regular users of primary care services.

A common problem to any marketing effort and a critical one in planning health service programs is the prediction of "sales," the estimation of how much utilization a given program can expect. For primary care programs involving people likely to have some current arrangement for handling their perceived needs, this is especially necessary.[26] If a hospital proposes to develop a new primary care center even in an area totally devoid of physicians, it must draw its customers from one or more of the following sources:

- People who now receive primary care from sources they may be willing to abandon in favor of a more accessible alternative.
- People who now use little or no primary care but would if a source were made available.
- Growth or migration which will produce more or different customers.

The easiest method of estimating the market would be to simply count noses and multiply each times some physician/population ratio. If it is assumed that there ought to be one physician per 2500 population, then a market area with 10,000 population and no physicians should presumably be able to support four physicians. A more complex calculation might include counting the population (e.g., 10,000 people), multiplying by an anticipated utilization rate (e.g., three visits per person per year) to yield total utilization (30,000 visits), then dividing by some expected productivity level per physician (e.g., 6000 visits per year) to yield physician requirements (in this case $30,000 \div 6000 = 5$ physicians).

Neither of these calculations guarantees that if four or five physicians are suddenly plunked down in the area they will immediately attract the utilization expected. The local population may have strong attachments to their current sources of care, even though quite a distance away. The trip to a distant physician may include the opportunity to visit relatives, do some shopping, get away from the dreary local surroundings or otherwise offer substantial secondary benefits. Should the existing patterns of care persist, the new program may well prove a disaster, benefiting neither the local community nor the hospital.

Approaching the Market

The marketing discipline offers many potentially useful concepts and techniques for primary care program development. Because the hospital is trying to "market" a service directly to the customer (patient), the primary care situation is very much analogous to traditional marketing situations. It is likely that most, if not all of the following techniques of approaching the market can be useful:

- **Identify and measure** exactly what the consumer needs from primary care. The "utilities" of such care include: relief from anxiety, relief from pain, protection from illness, etc.
- **Analyze current responses** available in the event of such needs. The "competition" may include non-medical providers such as pharmacists, chiropractors, faith healers, etc., as well as physicians in distant areas. Determine the utilities vs. costs of such responses from the consumer perspective.
- **Decide the feasibility and desirability of responding to unmet needs** given the hospital's financial, personnel and other resources.
- **Determine the potential for attracting patients** willing and able to pay (out-of-pocket, private health insurance, Medicare, Medicaid, etc.) what the hospital has determined to be requisite charges for services.
- **Identify specific market segments** which may be particularly attractive in terms of potential utilization and payment or which may require a separate product, price, place or promotion. Characteristics such as income, education, location, ethnic identity, health status, age, etc., may suggest separate treatment in some phase of program development.
- **Design the services, locations, hours of operation, facilities, personnel, equipment, etc., most appropriate to the "markets"** identified.
- **Determine which services the organization is best suited to provide, are most likely to succeed.**
- **Decide on the "price" for such services,** including all that potential patients must go through in order to utilize them. This

includes not only out-of-pocket payment but waiting for appointments, waiting to be seen, travel to the site of care, loss of time from work, type of personal handling by program staff, etc. All such "costs" must be balanced by the benefit or utilities of the services provided, and contrasted to competitive offerings.

- **Implement and adjust the program,** evaluating its results and correcting its shortcomings from both organizational and patient perspectives.

Specific marketing techniques, such as market research, financial feasibility analysis, segmenting markets, market analysis, communication, etc., are likely to be useful in such efforts. Techniques developed and tested in marketing manufactured products of all kinds will have to be modified somewhat in marketing health services. However, to ignore the potential of such techniques risks two major consequences:

1. The development of new programs using only traditional non-marketing design (this is what we want to do, come get it) may prove unsuccessful, resulting in the wrong product at the wrong place at the wrong price without effective promotion. This may mean either failure of the program, extensive additional cost in adjusting the program after the fact, or at least, less than optimal results.
2. The organization failing to employ effective marketing principles and techniques may lose out to the competition. Those health care institutions which market well are very likely to do better than those which market less well or not at all.

The development of new health services as well as the success of existing programs is important enough to work at doing well. While increasing regulation of health organizations makes innovation more difficult, it is still worth avoiding failure.[27] Marketing comprises the design and management of transactions between providers and consumers which satisfy both.[28] Given this definition there should be no objection to marketing health services in principle. Given the effectiveness of marketing in other areas, those health organizations which learn to employ marketing principles and methods effectively stand to benefit, as do the communities they serve.

REFERENCES

1. Kotler, P. and Zaltman, G. "Social Marketing: An Approach to Planned Social Change." *Journal of Marketing* 35:3 (July 1971) p. 3.

2. *Ibid.*

3. Kotler, P. *Marketing for Nonprofit Organizations* (Englewood Cliffs, N.J.: Prentice-Hall 1975) Ch. 16.

4. Zaltman, G. and Vertinsky, I. "Health Service Marketing: A Suggested Model." *Journal of Marketing* 35:3 (July 1971) p. 19.

5. Crane, R. *et al.* "The Marketing of Medical Care Services." Ch. 10 in ed. *Marketing in the Service Sector.* J. M. Rathmell, ed. (Cambridge, Mass.: Winthrop Publishers 1974).

6. Kotler, P. "A Generic Concept of Marketing." *Journal of Marketing* 36:2 (April 1972) p. 46.

7. Crane, R. "Marketing of Medical Care Services." p. 180.

8. Urban, G. "Ideas on a Decision Information System for Family Planning." *Industrial Management Review* 10 (Spring 1969) p. 45.

9. Hutchinson, J. "Using TV to Recruit Family Planning Patients." *Family Planning Perspectives* 2 (March 1970).

10. Farley, J. and Leavitt, H. "Marketing and Population Problems." *Journal of Marketing* 35:3 (July 1971) p. 28.

11. El-Ansary, A. and Kramer, O. "Social Marketing: The Family Planning Experience." *Journal of Marketing* 37:3 (July 1973) p. 1.

12. Berelson, B. "The Present State of Family Planning Programs." *Studies in Family Planning* 57 (September 1970) p. 8.

13. Ball, D. "An Abortion Clinic Ethnography" in *Qualitative Methodology.* W. J. Filstead, ed. (Chicago, Ill.: Markham Publishing 1970).

14. Burke, R. *Guidelines for HMO Marketing* (Minneapolis, Minn.: Interstudy 1973).

15. Mindak, W. and Bybee, H. "Marketing's Application to Fund-Raising." *Journal of Marketing* 35:3 (July 1971) p. 13.

16. Fink, R. *et al.* "Impact of Efforts to Increase Participation in Repetitive Screenings for Early Breast Cancer Detection." *American Journal of Public Health* (March 1972) p. 328.

17. Katz, T. and Soigir, M. "Effects of Souvenir Giveaways on Response to Offers of Free Chest X-Rays." *Public Health Reports* (August 1967) p. 735.

18. Walker, J. *et al.* "An Experimental Program in Ambulatory Medical Care." *New England Journal of Medicine* 271 (July 9, 1964) p. 63.

19. O'Halloran, R. *et al.* "Marketing Your Hospital." *Hospital Progress* (December 1976) p. 68.

20. Announced in *Hospital Week.* (November 16, 1974).

21. Olendzki, M. "The Present Role of the Community Hospital in Primary Ambulatory Care." Ch. 4 in *Community Hospitals and the Challenge of Primary Care* (New York: Columbia University Center for Community Health Systems 1975) p. 55.

22. Lincoln, J. "Development of a Satellite Family Health Center." *Medical Care* 12:3 (March 1974) p. 260.

23. *Ibid.* p. 264.

24. Simpson, J. "The Ashland Plan: An Ambulatory Care Outreach Alternative for a Community Hospital." *Hospital Administration* 20:3 (Summer 1975) p. 33.

25. "Chicago Hospital Announces Plans for Satellite Clinics." *Hospitals, J.A.H.A.* 48 (November 16, 1974).

26. Luft, H. *et al.* "Factors Affecting the Use of Physician Services in a Rural Community." *American Journal of Public Health* 66:9 (September 1976) p. 865.

27. Tauber, E. "Reduce New Product Failures: Measure Needs as Well as Purchases Interest." *Journal of Marketing* 37:3 (July 1973) p. 61.

28. Kotler, P. *Marketing for Non-Profit Organization* p. 5.

CONSIDERATION (OR PRICING) FOR SERVICES

INTRODUCTION

In marketing in the business sector, consideration is referred to as pricing. If the business marketing sector approach were to be transferred directly to the health care sector, it probably would be translated into rate setting. The issue is much more complex. The key concept behind marketing is consumer satisfaction and, unfortunately, that concept usually is sidestepped even in business in favor of the demand/supply considerations in business economics. In many courses on business sector marketing, the issue of the psychological side of pricing is stressed. It suggests that it is possible to raise the price and, instead of expecting to find a decrease in demand, to see an increase. Consumer perception of quality or prestige may enter into the phenomenon. The opposite may occur also (drop the price and demand drops) for similar reasons.

In this section the two selections, "Price of Services" and "Does This Patient Have a Real Beef," go beyond the issue of the price and rates to elements of value to consumers that they give up in exchange for health care services. For example, it includes the "price" one pays for waiting, inconsideration, discomfort, personal interaction, etc.

14. Price of Services

ROBIN E. MACSTRAVIC

Reprinted from *Marketing Health Care*, Chapter 12, pages 171–181, by permission of Aspen Systems Corporation, © 1977.

In the normal context of *price,* we usually mean the out-of-pocket payment of money expected in return for receipt of a given product or service. In the health services area, however, this is likely to be an overly restricted conception of price. In the first place, health insurance or government programs have eliminated or reduced direct, out-of-pocket payments by patients. Moreover, physicians are likely to make most determinations of which services will be used by a patient, so the price to the patient may not enter. Finally, the cost to the patient of using a given service vs. not using it, or receiving it through another organization, involves a great deal more than payment of money, even where that is necessary.

The notion of price in a market transaction is that which the consumer exchanges in return for what he receives. The payment of money is the obvious thing exchanged and the one which the provider gets in return for rendering the service. Thus, traditional marketing has focused on the cost to the consumer that becomes return to the provider. However, the decision by the potential consumer involves all the benefits he perceives vs. all the costs he perceives rather than merely the obvious service itself and its price tag in money.

The potential patient is likely to view cost or price as comprising everything he has to go through in order to receive the services he or his physician has determined are needed. For some services, this cost may include, but is rarely limited to, the direct payment of money from his pocket. In addition, he may be expected to transport himself from the place where the need arises to where the service is offered (Nobody makes house calls anymore!). He may have to wait hours, days, or weeks to get an appointment. Even after arriving for an appointment, he may have to wait minutes or hours to be seen. He may put up with impersonal treatment, uncomfortable diagnostic procedures, and painful treatment. All these are best examined as costs to the patient if they influence his choice as to whether and from whom to utilize specific services.

MONEY

The price paid in money by the patient may serve a number of purposes. First, of course, it represents income to the organization. The prospect of such income may have played a vital role in deciding whether or not to offer a specific service. Additionally, the price may be taken as a measure of quality. The high-priced physician, hospital, or nursing home may be taken by the public to be the high quality provider. We tend to value services according to what we pay for them, so charges may be necessary lest we consider services worthless. Moreover, price may serve a rationing function, preventing people who don't really need a given service from trying to use it. One of the great fears of eliminating out-of-pocket payments for health services has been the feeling that people would demand all sorts of services unnecessarily.

Money considerations also have varied impact on the offering of a specific service. The organization may determine what price to charge for a service requiring out-of-pocket payment on the basis of what it costs the organization to provide the service. Recalling the law of supply and demand, however, unless demand for the service is completely inelastic to price, different amounts of the service may tend to be utilized at different price levels. Thus the break-even analysis described previously may have to be repeated at different price levels because of the different utilization levels they would be expected to achieve.

In general, there are three common approaches for deciding what monetary price to charge for a given service, all occasionally used in pricing health services. The pricing practice most common in health care is cost-based pricing, where price is determined on the basis of mark-up over unit cost. To some extent, demand-based pricing is also possible, where price is set to what the market will bear. A third option is competition-based pricing, where prices are set so as to be roughly equal to what others are charging.

Cost-based pricing may seem the fairest form of price determination since it most clearly aims at making the exchange transaction equitable to the health organization. Costs of services should be relatively simple to ascertain, though different indirect cost allocation procedures may be followed by different organizations. Cost-based pricing avoids taking advantage of the patient in need of care, while being fair to the provider. On the other hand, one organization's costs may be unnecessarily high because of its inefficiency or low volume of utilization. If a given charge would make utilization prohibitive, it may not be possible to cover costs if the competition offers similar services at substantially lower prices.

Demand-based pricing may not seem fair in that it seemingly takes advantage of the extent of need and demand for a given health service. Frequently, however, demand based pricing may be used in an attempt to alter the timing or level of demand. The high price charged for emergency department care is not determined by its price, but is designed to discourage use for nonemergency conditions. Lower prices may be charged for ambulatory surgery in an effort to shift utilization away from inpatient care. Theoretically, lower charges could be made on weekends in an attempt to smooth out daily variations in demand. For this to work, of course, both physicians and patients as determiners of the timing of utilization, must feel the effects of price differences. This is often not the case.

In general, demand-based pricing may be necessary to make up for the limits of cost-reimbursement formulas for many types of health services. The hospital may develop new services with the specific intention that they be sources of charge-based rather than cost reimbursement. Only by having some such sources can the organization hope to make up for bad debts when most services are cost reimbursed.

Competition-based pricing is part of the reality of most health services pricing. A health organization must be sensitive to what others are charging for similar services, even when the consumer doesn't pay the charge directly. It is probably not considered good public relations to charge significantly more for the same services as similar organizations in the same area. Conversely, in some cases, a higher charge may be considered an indication of higher quality care or amenities, and hence attract patients. Where patients pay charges directly, as in primary care programs, hospitals may find it necessary to set charges equivalent to those of private physicians.

In practice, determination of price level is likely to exhibit some aspects of all three approaches. Where possible, the health organization is likely to attempt to set its charges above its cost per unit of service, so that a given service program might pay its own way. In order to discourage unnecessary utilization or adjust the timing or intensity of demand, it may gear prices to demand levels. It may do the same in order to make up for services where costs cannot be recovered. In any case, it is necessary to be aware of competition pricing, if only for the public relations effects.

TRANSPORTATION

The difficulty encountered in getting to the source of care is another example of cost to the patient, but a cost that is not directly translated into benefits to the institution. There are indirect benefits, however. The patient's coming to the provider enables the provider to see more patients. This in turn may be reflected in lower charges to the patient, so the effects work both ways. The question of access in terms of time or distance may become critical in some situations. Emergency medical services are one area where attempts have been made to get care to the patient in the shortest possible time, rather than merely to get the patient to [the] care.

In designing a specific strategy for achieving a desired utilization from a given market, the organization may develop any of a number of approaches to transportation components of patient costs. A given service may be offered at a number of fixed or mobile sites in order to maximize access. Storefronts, church basements, and mobile vans have all been used at various times by different health organizations. In many cases, outreach workers may be employed to go out and bring the patient to care, or public transportation may be paid for.

In examining the utilization transaction from the patient's perspective, the health organization ought to view transportation as a part of the price it expects patients to pay, even though it doesn't receive the income. In making site selections, the organization may be able to locate an area central to travel routes and movement patterns with positive impact on both utilization and patient satisfaction. The organization may have to counter each incremental increase in transportation difficulty with a service benefit to achieve or maintain utilization levels it desires.

HOURS

The hours in which given health services are offered have substantial impact on the price patients pay for care. Where services are available only during normal working hours, many people may be seriously inconvenienced or even lose money. The mother may have to locate and even pay for a baby sitter, or bring her children with her to get care she or a child requires. Working people may lose wages for each hour they miss from work. Depending on the time of an appointment, patients may have to worm their way through rush hour traffic in crowded urban areas.

Hours may be easier to adjust in theory than in practice, however. Since the medical staff and employees are likely to prefer normal working hours, the organization may be locked into these traditional hours of operation. To achieve desired utilization levels, however, some adjustment may be necessary. If inconvenience and loss of income prevent people from using services, or lead them to select more convenient providers, new balances in the utilization transaction may be required. The "price" which different hours of service availability generates may determine utilization, especially of services for which the patient initiates contact.

WAITING

Delays in receiving health services may arise in two ways. In the first place, there may be a substantial wait before a patient can get an appointment. For relatively elective services such as routine check-ups or minor symptoms, such delays might be acceptable. For others, they may result in delays past the optimal point for providing care or cause prospective patients to seek care elsewhere. An organization obviously can't be sure to have appointment times available every day, for that would mean it is operating well below capacity. At the same time, rigid adherence to appointment limits may cause loss of regular patients and result in unused capacity in the long run.

The second and often most onerous type of delay is the waiting room wait. Here, too, organizational efficiency may dictate that patients must wait so that physicians and other professionals don't have to. On the other hand, the wait is a cost to the patient that may in the long run result in lost patients. By not creating too many appointments at the beginning of the day, by starting to see patients on time and trying to stick to its own schedule, the organization may minimize unnecessary waiting time and increase patient satisfaction.

DISCOMFORT

Health care in most cases is likely to involve some patient discomfort, dysfunction, or pain. Much of this is unavoidable, but some may result from indifference. Substantial efforts have been made to make relatively elective services such as immunization shots as painless as possible. Surgery and filling teeth can be relatively painless, though rarely enjoyable. Frequently, however, bothersome discomforts remain, if only because they may appear minor to the provider, though not necessarily to the patient.

If the providers of health services could occasionally experience what patients do, some changes might take place in health care delivery. Do patients really have to be clothed in backless and virtually bottomless hospital pajamas? Do they have to be woken (*sic*) at midnight to take a sleeping pill, at 6:00 a.m. to have breakfast before they're hungry? Do they really have to be left in corridors waiting for lab tests or x-rays, or until the transport aide gets around to taking them where they're supposed to go?

Some discomforts may truly be necessary. A barium enema or proctoscopy can hardly be carried out in a thoroughly dignified manner. So too, some discomfort may be psychologically necessary, as when people think medicine must taste bad to be effective. As with access difficulties, however, discomfort is part of the price the patient pays for care. Where the price becomes too high in comparison to the perceived benefits, or where a competitor offers a better deal, such a price may result in loss of patients' utilization, however necessary it might be.

PERSONAL INTERACTIONS

The aspect of health care which most markedly differs from most other services is the impersonality of human interaction which so often accompanies it. Clerks in retail establishments, salespeople in general, and people whose jobs require pleasing customers are selected and trained for high quality personal interactions. Health care delivery has somehow divorced itself from the intensity of concern over client wishes that prevails in most exchange transactions. The health system is not unique in this regard, of course. Many governmental agencies act as if they're doing clients a favor rather than attracting mutually beneficial exchanges.

Contrasts between ward and private patients, between the attitudes shown private pay vs. Medicaid patients, or whites vs. blacks, or any discrimination between different types of patients is likely to be viewed as an oppressive price by the disadvantaged, though perhaps as an added benefit by the advantaged. The individual organization which is successful in dealing with the personal needs and sensitivities of its clients is likely to be successful in other ways as well.

SUMMARY

In general, the price the patient is expected to pay for services rendered includes much more than money. To design and execute effective market strategies, the health organization must be able to identify and weigh all the things a patient must go through as costs to actual or prospective patients which must balance perceived benefits for desired utilization to occur. Health services may be relatively inelastic to money price where need for care is emergent and no out-of-pocket charge is made. Their utilization may well be elastic to other price forms, however. The health organization which can identify and achieve improvements in the price exchange relationship is likely to be able to achieve the levels and types of utilization it wishes.

All parts of service design are likely to affect the price people pay for health services in the largest sense. Attributes of service form, such as convenience of use, safety, side-effects, and interference with normal functioning all involve costs to the patient. Attributes of service organization and delivery, such as fragmentation of care and difficulty in getting to the source of care and finding a place to park also require the patient to spend himself in return for health services. The formal price in money as well as transportation, time-loss, waiting, impersonal care, etc. are further demands placed on the patient who seeks an organization's services.

Since all these represent costs to the patient, the health organization must ensure that benefits to the patient are commensurate. This may involve carefully explaining to each patient exactly what the benefits are in ways he can understand. In many cases this will not be sufficient. To achieve desired utilization levels, the health organization should be prepared to manage the costs it places between the prospective patient and receipt of care in the same way it manages the delivery of such care. It is not only proper that health organizations do so, but is likely to be a practical necessity as competition for patient transactions increases in the future.

15. Does this Patient Have a Real Beef?

SUSAN M. WERSHING

Reprinted by permission from the February 23, 1976 issue of *Medical Economics*, copyright © 1976 by Litton Industries, Inc. Published by Medical Economics Company, a Litton Division, at Oradell, NJ 07649.

If you have days when you're way behind on your appointment schedule and feeling harassed about it, it's a good bet that patients cooling their heels in your waiting room are fully as unhappy. At a time when antidoctor sentiment is on the rise—and malpractice suits along with it—this is one of the commonest patient complaints.

You may not realize just how common it is, because most patients can't bring themselves to complain to the doctor; they simply sound off to their families and friends. So you may not be doing anything to mollify patients when you have to keep them waiting an hour or more.

Every so often a patient who goes through such an experience *does* make an issue of it. Not long ago the mother of a patient in Wheaton, Md., contacted *Medical Economics* and asked if there was anything we could do to bring this problem home to our doctor-readers. We suggested that she first try to get satisfaction through local channels, beginning with a letter to her doctor, and keep us posted. Tempering her indignation, she wrote the physician.

March 25, 1975

Dear Dr. _____ :

I am writing to describe a recent experience at your office that upset me greatly.

Approximately one month in advance, I made an appointment for my 12-year-old daughter to be examined by you. I explained that I would have to take leave from work and would appreciate an appointment as late in the day as possible. Your secretary made a very strong point that 3 p.m. was the latest slot you would schedule, and so it was set. She asked for my home and office telephone numbers in case she needed to do any rescheduling for your convenience.

The day of the appointment, I arranged for my daughter to be dismissed early from school, and with my husband—we share one car—took several hours off from work. We traveled approximately 30 miles—from our office to the school, and then to your office—arriving tired but on time. Then we sat and we waited—for fully an hour and a half.

While I waited, the receptionist handed me a form so I could provide information establishing that I was able to pay the bill. But absolutely no effort was made by the appointment secretaries, the medical assistant, or yourself to explain that there would be a long delay—much less to apologize for its necessity. Occasionally I checked the time at the secretaries' desk. Behind it was a wall plaque warning me that cancellations must be made by the patient 24 hours in advance to avoid a charge for the appointment.

Around 4:10, your medical assistant moved us from the waiting room to an examination room, giving rise to a false hope that the examination was imminent.

At 4:30, I told your secretary I was leaving. She made no comment. I then went to your study in a pretty angry state and told you I was leaving, and why. Either because you were not interested in going into the matter or were taken aback by my strong feelings, you said nothing to suggest you thought the situation was unfortunate or in any way regrettable. You simply nodded your head goodby. Perhaps it was the last straw in *your* day.

I appreciate the possibility of an emergency arising. This may be a frequent occurrence in some types of practice. Anyone can have an emergency (although your wall plaque makes no allowances for any but yours). However, your secretary had my telephone number. She could have phoned me at my office to say there would be a delay, and we could have altered our schedules accordingly. I honestly believe the reason she didn't phone is that neither you nor your assistants ever thought of it, because doctors' practices are scheduled exclusively for *their* convenience. In this regard, I know of no other business situation where the seller expresses such a total disinterest in and contempt for the buyer.

Perhaps I should have come to the appointment wearing my own plaque, warning that the cost of delay beyond a 15-minute period would be deducted from the bill. Laughable? I estimate that this visit, which was a total waste, cost me and my husband the equivalent in leave time of $70, not to mention the gas used in traveling.

So far I've put the matter in business terms—money lost, time lost. But what I most resented was the indifference that prompted me to leave. Whatever the cause of the delay, if at any point someone had expressed awareness that we had been waiting too long and asked for our tolerance, I would not be writing this letter.

Patients are people, not body counts. When doctors become aware their appointments will be backed up, they should instruct their secretaries to phone affected patients and advise them of the delay. If this is not possible, the secretaries should tell the patients when they arrive that there will be a delay and make a simple apology for the inconvenience. This is normal courtesy and costs nothing.

Finally, a doctor who, because of the nature of his practice, cannot rely on meeting his appointments promptly, should not demand cancellation notices 24 hours in advance. What per cent of gross income is represented by charges for canceled appointments? I doubt it's worth the ill will it must cause. People who make the decision to call for appointments do not generally do so for frivolous reasons, and if they are prevented from keeping the appointment because of an emergency, it's likely the emergency arose in less than 24 hours. The patient, of course, owes the doctor the courtesy of a phone cancellation as soon as possible. For the few patients who chronically cancel appointments, the doctor has the sensible alternative of suggesting that they seek medical attention elsewhere.

I close with the hope that you will respond to this letter with concern. If you have any comments, I would very much appreciate hearing them.

Sincerely yours,
(Mrs.) Adelaide Edelson

If the doctor had acknowledged that she had a point, and had promised to try harder to spare patients such inconvenience in the future, that would have ended the matter. But Mrs. Edelson heard nothing. After a month she called us again. We next suggested that she take her complaint to the local medical society.

She sent them a copy of her original letter, along with a note asking if they had "any policy on the issues raised in the letter." On May 5 she received a standard acknowledgment, stating that her letter was in the hands of the society's Professional Relations Committee, and that she would hear from them when the review was completed.

Another two months went by before Mrs. Edelson received this official communication:

July 13, 1975

Montgomery County Medical Society
2446 Reedie Drive, Wheaton, Maryland 20902
Re: Case No. C–45–251

Dear Mrs. Edelson:

The Professional Relations Committee of the Montgomery County Medical Society has made a thorough investigation of your complaint concerning the inordinate time you and your husband waited with your daughter in Dr. _____'s office. Dr. _____ states that on the day in question he had a number of unexpected delays occasioned by his having to spend longer periods of time with patients than he had anticipated. The nature of these delays, of course, did not permit him to make advance alterations in his afternoon schedule. Dr. _____ regrets the inconvenience caused you and your family and offers his apologies with the hope that you obtained satisfactory medical attention elsewhere. He would have liked to have extended these in person had you not left his office so hastily.

We hope this provides a satisfactory solution to your complaint.

Sincerely yours,

The letter, signed by the chairman of the Professional Relations Committee, was *not* "a satisfactory solution" to Mrs. Edelson. While it gave an explanation of the delay and conveyed the other doctor's apology, it ignored her complaint that at no point had the doctor or his assistants "expressed awareness that we had been waiting too long and asked for our tolerance."

At this stage *Medical Economics* began looking into the situation. We first phoned Dr. _____ , an orthopedist in a five-man practice, to get his version of the incident.

Did he remember a patient's mother named Adelaide Edelson? "Yes, I wrote a reply to that to the county."

Why hadn't he answered her letter? "I think I was away when the letter came in."

Do delays like that happen all the time? "In an orthopedic practice they happen quite frequently, yes. If you get someone who comes in with an acute injury, we'll do them first, rather than the patient sitting in the office."

Has he done anything to reduce patient waiting times, such as having an assistant make adjustments in the schedule when she saw he was running behind? "How can you do that? It's impossible. You can't. Look, you're interrupting me now. You're keeping my patients waiting in the office now."

Our next call was to the chairman of the Professional Relations Committee of the county medical society. His society participates in such public service projects as a telephone service to help newcomers find doctors. There are plenty of newcomers in Montgomery County. Composed of bedroom communities outside Washington, D.C., it's the fourth biggest county in the state, with a population of well over 500,000. Of its 1,770 doctors, some 1,100 belong to the county society.

We asked the professional relations chairman what kind of investigation his committee made when it got a complaint from a patient.

"We write to the physician, provide him with a copy of the correspondence, and ask him to reply," he said. "Then we review the answer. If we're not satisfied, we pursue it further. But in this case, the doctor was quite apologetic."

He acknowledged that there had been other complaints about Dr. _____ , but said they had nothing to do with making patients wait. "In fact, that's the only letter of complaint we've had with regard to waiting in a physician's office in the entire three years that I've been on the committee."

Says Mrs. Edelson: "I showed my letter to some people at work, and did *that* open the floodgates!"

What of Dr. _____'s contention that it's impossible to avoid waiting-room delays? "It happens in my own office," the committee chairman said. "You give me 10:30 in the morning, and I'm an hour behind. And when I find someone who's really upset because he's had to wait an hour and a half, I tell him we do our best. If he feels it's really too much, I ask if he'd like the names of a couple of doctors who might schedule differently."

As long as this attitude persists among physicians, they're courting patient-relations trouble—or worse. In Mrs. Edelson's case, her daughter had been having pains in her knee, probably stemming from her activity in school sports. "She was suffering so much, I finally inquired around, and this doctor had such a good reputation, especially with sports injuries, I decided it was worth the trip." Did she go to another doctor afterward? "No, I was so disgusted, I ignored the problem, and it went away."

Suppose it hadn't?

ACCESS TO HEALTH CARE

INTRODUCTION

As noted in the introduction to this section, there is a need to avoid direct transference of marketing to the health care sector from the business (or goods) sector. This section describes specific areas for marketing's contribution in health care, concentrating on access and availability issues in health care marketing. In the business sector this is referred to as the "place," or the element of marketing management that concentrates on the distribution of the product. Distribution includes transportation, inventory control, warehousing, etc.

It has been pointed out frequently in this book that consumer orientation and satisfaction are the focus and keystone of the marketing concept. Ironically, the health care terms of "access" and "availability" (chosen for this section) contain a greater notion of consumer orientation than the traditional marketing term of "place" or distribution.

The two readings chosen to illustrate consumer orientation in access and availability are "Users Point the Way to Best Hospital Design" and "A Mobile Resource for Senior Citizens." The first article, on hospital design (which dates back to 1969), was chosen for two reasons: first, it illustrates that bits and pieces of what now is called health care marketing have existed for a long time; and secondly, it describes how a hospital's administrators obtained, through market testing, patient and staff input to design a hospital addition.

The second article is an original manuscript describing the evaluation of an innovative health delivery system in which the distribution aspects play the key role. It is a clear example of consumer orientation based not on what others thought senior citizens wanted but on a clear understanding of how the target market was responding to previously offered services.

16. Users Point Way to Best Hospital Design

ROBERT BYRNE

Reprinted from *Modern Hospital* by permission of Crain Communications, © November 1969.

Market testing—a technique that consumer products manufacturers use to discover the reactions of the public before full-scale manufacturing and distribution—has been adapted by Providence Memorial Hospital, El Paso, Tex., to the planning of its 132 bed addition. The result is an efficient and pleasing structure.

During the early stages of construction planning, Providence officials called in nurses and physicians to find out what the people working on the nursing floors wanted in patient room layouts and equipment. Then, three mock-ups were built, the first based on the staff's comments and the others on successive suggested changes. Even some patients were brought to the mock-up rooms to uncover user attitudes.

Later, planners went to a local high school's fieldhouse to lay out a full-scale patient floor. Nurses and doctors then were able to walk through the proposed arrangement and recommend any changes in sizes or layout. A similar procedure was followed in the planning of the operating rooms to be included in the new building.

One reason for the elaborate preparations was the difficulty of designing an appropriate addition to the original X-shaped building. The result of the planning and testing is a rectangular tower that connects two arms of the X shape. The buildings are joined by long glassed-in corridors that lead from the midsection of the addition to the junction of the wings of the X.

The new building, which was opened about two years ago, is constructed of reinforced concrete, with concrete slab and face brick on the exterior to match the appearance of the existing hospital building.

After the addition was completed, remodeling was begun in the older building. Total capacity of the hospital was raised to 430 beds.

A circular driveway was built around the entire hospital during the construction of the addition. Previously, many patients had to be discharged through the emergency entrance because of the long walk from the main entrance to the street.

Patient rooms, to which so much time and planning effort was devoted, are 16 feet 3 inches by 10 feet 8 inches. The bed in each room is set at an angle to the outside wall. Alongside the bed and projecting out from the side wall are the lavatory and service cabinets. This ar-

Figure 1 Ground Floor Plan

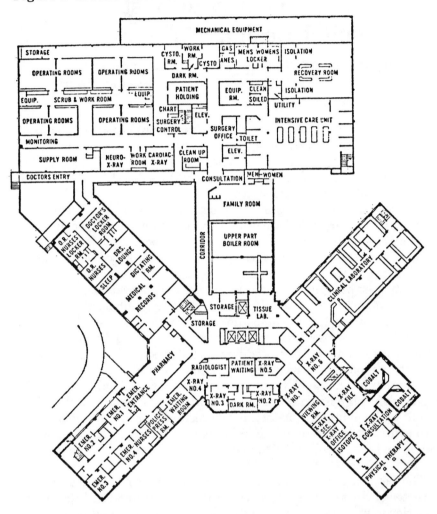

Note: Ground floor of addition houses surgical and intensive care facilities. Addition is connected to main building, where emergency department, pharmacy, and x-ray are located, by long corridor and family room.

---

rangement makes it possible for a patient to sit on the foot of his bed while using the lavatory. The bedside console also includes telephone, running ice water, switches for mirror and reading lights, TV and radio controls, and the nurse call system.

Each of the private rooms contains its own toilet and shower enclosure. Instead of conventionally locating this space along the corridor, the Providence plan places the washroom on the outside wall, behind the patient's bed position. This required protrusions into the exterior wall, but the architects turned this to an advantage since it provided a means of breaking up the flat surfaces of the tower.

Lighting for the patient's bed is provided by two bullet lights, one at the head of the bed that serves as a reading light and the other at the foot of the bed. When both lights are on, there is more than sufficient illumination for examinations and treatment. The light over the foot of the bed is controlled by a dimmer switch at the doorway, so a night nurse can enter quietly and turn the light up just enough to check the patient's condition without disturbing his sleep.

Because of the bed's angle, patients are able to look out through the window while lying back. The windows are double-pane with venetian blinds between panes for sun control. Windows are mounted on pivots so that the outside pane can be turned into the room for washing.

Rooms are decorated in color schemes of yellow, blue or green, and walls are ornamented with framed prints. The broad corridors are painted light colors and equipped with handrails.

The four nursing floors in the addition are virtually identical. Each floor is arranged in the double-corridor, racetrack design with nurses' stations and supply spaces located in the center and patient rooms laid against the outside walls.

The bottom or basement level of the addition actually is above ground because of the site's slope. This level is connected to the basement of the older building through a newly constructed laundry.

Food service facilities, storage areas, and the central service department are located in the basement level of the addition. The central service is linked to the surgical area on the floor immediately above by two dumbwaiters, one for sterile goods and the other for dirty equipment and supplies.

Surgical suites, including x-ray-equipped rooms for cardiac and neurological surgery, are on the ground floor level. Also located here are two cystoscopy rooms, the 16 bed intensive care unit, and the 18 bed recovery room. The corridor connecting this area to the corresponding level in the older building contains a family room or lounge. In this position, the room is near the emergency, laboratory and x-ray rooms of the original building as well as the facilities in the addition.

The eight new operating rooms in the addition are arranged around a central scrub and work area. Both the recovery room and the I.C.U. use island-type nursing stations. Two beds in the recovery unit are in cubicles that allow for isolation cases; all beds in the I.C.U. are private.

Although the four nursing floors are basically alike, the first nursing level includes an occupational therapy room which is accessible through the connecting corridor to the psychiatric unit in the older building. Every nursing floor includes a classroom, nurses' lounge, head nurse's office, and a small family lounge.

The nurses' station on each floor is located in front of the two passenger elevators . . . .

According to Providence officials, patients and staff have expressed satisfaction with the features of the new structure. Administrators feel this positive reaction is, to a great extent, the result of giving everyone a chance to help plan the facility rather than waiting for the complaints to surface after the addition was built.

17. A Mobile Resource for Older Persons

KEMSEY J. MACKEY AND MINDY ZINN

Adapted by the authors from an article originally published in *Hospitals, Journal of the American Hospital Association*, Vol. 52, January 1, 1978. Copyright 1978, American Hospital Association.

Introduction

In the spring of 1977 Saint Clare's Hospital, Denville, New Jersey, incorporated into its mental health services an innovative and unique way to provide services to the senior citizen population of Morris County, New Jersey. A mobile drop-in center travels throughout the county stopping at pre-arranged sites and provides a variety of services to anyone over the age of 60. A community mental health nurse, a mental health counselor/driver and a social worker provide informal health and mental health counseling, hypertensive and audiometric screening, and information and referral in a warm and friendly environment.

An article entitled "Mobile Center Links Providers with Isolated Senior Citizens" by M. R. Stuart and K. J. Mackey[1] explained in detail the historic perspective and developmental milestones of this program. However, since the program's inception, significant changes have occurred. The acquisition of a new vehicle, changes in staffing, schedule and site rearrangements and funding are some of the areas where alterations have taken place. These programmatic changes have had a positive impact on the population receiving services.

In order to fully understand this program as it now exists an examination of the evolutionary process is essential to understanding its present status. Therefore, this article will focus on the history, growth and future projections of this mobile outreach project and its effect on the senior citizens of Morris County.

The Mobile Drop-In Center is an effective and viable alternative for increasing awareness and delivering services in the fields of physical and mental health care. Health care professionals are often unable to reach these older persons who need concrete service, such as physical therapy, nutrition guidance, medication counseling, hypertension screening and counseling and referrals to other appropriate resources. Moreover, the underserviced, isolated older person frequently has a number of emotional difficulties which go unattended since he/she does not seek help from "traditional" sources. A mobile center reaching out to the older person replaces the established modes of intervention and lessens the perceived burden of the senior citizen going for help. From this perspective this project represents a concrete framework for other communities to mold a similar program.

Birth of the Program

The acknowledgement of the need for counseling and social services on an outreach basis, especially for older people, came from a number of independent sources. This helped lay the groundwork for this program. These sources are St. Clare's Hospital Mental Health Services, the Morris County Co-Op Committee and the "SCAN" Survey.

Saint Clare's Hospital, a 246 bed institution with both a church and community affiliation, has always been actively involved in outreach programs for older people. In early 1975, a community mental health center was established which continued and expanded outreach to senior citizens in the community. Consultation and Education services were offered to both the management and clients of the county nutrition sites.

At about the same time, the hospital's mental health outpatient department discovered that persons over the age of 60 did not avail themselves of mental health services, especially on a direct service basis. Senior citizens represented approximately 13 percent of the county population, yet never more than 2–1/2 percent were included in the mental health center's active caseload. These statistics caused concern, especially considering the generally accepted fact that senior citizens have both emotional and social adjustment difficulties, as well as physical problems. Moreover, very often older people experience a number of problems simultaneously, which demand attention.

It was apparent that older people do not see themselves as needing psychiatric services even when emotional symptoms are present. Instead, they are concerned with housing, finances, abandonment, physical deterioration along with a loss of independence, and mobility. Very often older people are unable to cope with these problems, and so they withdraw and become socially isolated. On the other hand, senior citizens who are (or become) active in the community, maintain a more positive self image and exhibit signs of emotional and physical well-being. Therefore, it seemed essential that the isolated elderly citizen had to be linked to the health care and social service systems.

The second group concerned with senior citizens was the Morris County Co-Op Committee. The Co-Op Committee, an advisory council to the community planner of the county Department on Aging, reached similar conclusions about the county's older population and supported the initial plans for the mobile drop-in center. The reluctance of senior citizens to seek mental health services was disturbing to the committee members as well. Both the committee members and the mental health outpatient department drew similar conclusions about why the target population did not seek help. Briefly, they were: (1) that there was a lack of awareness and information about the nature and benefit of mental health counseling services; (2) hospital-based mental health programs can be inaccessible to the aged, who often have limited ability to travel and restricted accessibility to transportation; (3) the perceived high cost of psychiatric care also keeps the elderly from seeking much needed services; (4) senior citizens often react to the stigma attached to using mental health care and also fear involuntary commitment. Clearly, older people do not perceive their need for, nor do they actively seek, mental health services. At the same time, few, if any, preventative measures are made, and this results in exacerbated or chronic problems for the older people with unmanageable difficulties.

Finally, Morris County College (in conjunction with the County Department on Aging as a consultant) conducted a survey to assess senior citizens' needs. The results indicated that services were underutilized by senior citizens because they were either unaware of the existence of services or not cognizant of their eligibility for them. Pockets of poverty, scarcity of social and medical services and physical isolation were all found in central geographic areas. Furthermore, nursing home residents and older people living in the community did not emerge with significantly different amounts or severity of problems. Therefore, it was concluded that with adequate community support systems, more senior citizens could remain in their homes and the community.

St. Clare's Hospital, as a result of the information from these three sources, applied to the county Department on Aging and requested federal funding under Title III of the Older Americans Act. The project, with specific emphasis on its mobile nature, was viewed as accomplishing many of the objectives set forth by each of the parties concerned.

An area still to be explored was the financial commitment of the hospital's board of trustees. The board voted to supply 25 percent of the needed funds, and, at about the same time, a camper was donated, which was to be designed for use as the mobile center.

The time span encompassing these transactions was less than three months, thereby attesting to the enthusiasm and commitment of all parties involved. The grant was subsequently approved in November 1976.[2]

PURPOSE

The Senior Citizens Mobile Drop-In Center exists to help senior citizens achieve optimal physical and emotional well being while engendering a sense of being a vital, contributing member of society. Because of the existing and emerging needs of older people, this program is flexible in that it allows for the changing demands for services. The basic tenets of the program are to decrease social isolation while increasing one's self esteem, to enable persons to maximize their influence in decisions concerning themselves, to provide a vital link in the network of support systems and to maintain persons in their homes or the communities where they feel most comfortable. The mobile van meets seniors where they live and in so doing establishes an atmosphere where these tenets can be developed through providing specific services.

METHOD

When the program was first initiated, a 23 foot van was redesigned and furnished to provide space for a group meeting room and a small counseling area. However, shortly after the program began, the van size in relation to program needs proved unworkable. From the outset, the individual counseling area was a much needed and demanded service. Initially, the space seemed adequate but staff soon learned that the individual counseling space was too small and confining. Moreover, the group space did not lend itself to individual counseling since it did not foster a sense of confidentiality. A van which was more versatile in its overall usages was crucial to the program's success. This present van, though instrumental in operationalizing the program, was 7 years old and had a limited life-time. A proposal for a new vehicle was written, submitted for funding and ultimately approved. This time the vehicle was bought new and was custom designed to meet the needs of the program. A schematic representation of the physical layout of the new van [appears on the next page].

Originally the van visited all 39 municipalities in the county to discover the areas most in need of services, to further publicize this new project, and to see senior citizens' reaction to and utilization of this program. Evaluation of the project's "success" and need produced a change from the original scheduling. These changes were determined by: 1) areas where services were scarce and the municipality had stated a need and requested our services; 2) population density of senior citizens in a municipality; 3) coordination of services with

Figure 1 Layout of Senior Citizens' Mobile Drop-In Center

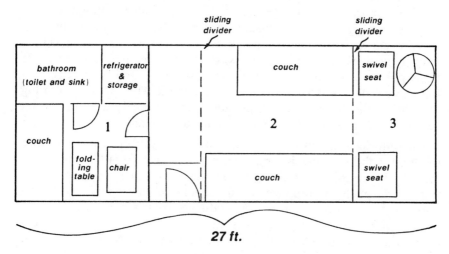

27 ft.

Note: Numbers 1, 2, and 3 represent areas where private counseling can occur.

municipal health and welfare departments attempting to avoid duplication of services; and, 4) geographic isolation of an area.

This assessment resulted in the elimination or reduction of visits to well serviced townships and the increase of visits to more need underserviced areas.

The new 27 foot van makes pre-arranged two hour stops, twice daily, in approximately 7 to 8 locations each week. Some sites are visited once a week, while other stops are made every two weeks and some are made once a month. The schedule remains very flexible. Special visits to places such as municipal health fairs, senior citizens clubs and nutrition sites, are often arranged and continually made upon request.

The actual site location in a given area was determined by ascertaining where senior citizens shop, bank, or spend their leisure time. Key persons (primarily municipal welfare officers) in each municipality provided this information. Most suggestions to the ideal stopping points were shopping centers, municipal buildings and downtown areas. Every town had one spot chosen that seemed accessible and familiar to the local senior citizen population.

Scope of Services

A wide range of social, medical, mental health and general supportive services are offered free of charge on the van. Both direct and indirect services are offered. The direct services, blood pressure checks and audiometric screening, are the most sought after services. These furnish a "portal of entry" to the van. As most older people are reluctant to openly seek mental health services, this direct aid provides a way in which the older person can request help without an open acknowledgement of need. Persons who clearly have perfect hearing or blood pressures often come to the van every week and request screening, have it done and remain on the van to talk. This "nonthreatening tool" helps the van staff reach persons who ordinarily would not seek services and who are in need of some kind of help.

The indirect services relate to health and mental health counseling frequently followed by information and referral. Health counseling includes helping senior citizens become aware of the names, doses and reasons for medication prescribed for them and advice on proper exercises, health maintenance and adequate nutrition. Counseling is given for any physical impairment resulting from the normal aging process or from an age related health problem such as glaucoma or heart disease.

On-the-spot, informal counseling is available in a relaxed environment where persons are encouraged to ventilate their feelings and/or concrete concerns. Seniors are invited to use all the time they need to talk about personal, medical or family problems. The private consultation area now available permits older persons to discuss their more intimate problems (financial, marital) with an increased sense of confidentiality. When difficulties arise that need further attention, the appropriate referral is made. However, the staff has noticed that older people most often hesitate to seek "traditional" mental health services. When this occurs, these persons are encouraged to come back to the van and to keep in touch by mail and phone.

Group discussions are also frequent events on the van with topics ranging from low salt cooking hints to common problems faced by older people (finances, abandonment, physical impairment, etc.). Structured formal educational programs and less formal spontaneous discussions are facilitated and encouraged by staff members. Peer discussions and resulting mutual support make seniors feel that their difficulties are not unique to them nor are they "different" because they are experiencing problems. They come to realize that many of their fears and feelings are shared by other persons as well. Visitors to the Drop-In Center are always encouraged to return and bring family or friends who also might benefit from this service. Everyone is encouraged to visit regularly and specific appointments for individuals or families are made upon request.

The van also contains a complete resource file with literature on federal, state and county programs available for older people. The staff is quite knowledgeable about these programs, and much effort is focused upon linking needy persons to the appropriate agency. Referrals are made and follow-up procedures are completed by van personnel and the agency involved. All referrals are closely monitored in order to guarantee effective follow-up on all visitors.

Vital information is recorded on all persons who visit. Demographic data includes: name, address, telephone number, marital status, health problems, notation of visits to the van, physicians' names, and comments on services provided. Visitors are also issued a card with this Project's name and telephone number, their name, and their physician's name. In addition, their blood pressures are recorded on this card and most carry it with them all the time.

Staff

As with many such projects, the Mobile Drop-In Van Program planned for a well balanced, multi-disciplined staff. The staff is composed of a Project Director (currently a mental health counselor), social worker, community mental health nurse, counselor/driver and a secretary. The Project Director supervises all field operations and personnel and is responsible for all publicity, policies and procedures, report writing and community liaison essential to the successful operation of this program. In addition, the director and social worker act as a consultant to the community and the community mental health center. The social worker also provides part time services on the van and spends additional time at various community agencies such as nutrition sites and senior clubs. The nurse performs health and mental health screening and counseling and is responsible for all medical information. The driver/counselor drives the van to the program sites, interacts with visitors and is responsible for follow-up on all referrals made. The secretary organizes and keeps all records. One of the Coordinators for mental health services at St. Clare's is involved with the Project and serves as an administrative resource person for the Project Director.

Funding

For the first two years of this program, funding came from the county Department on Aging through federal money allocated under Title III of the Older Americans Act in conjunction with Saint Clare's Hospital. However, St. Clare's Hospital is now able to operate the program through resources collected in other mental health departments, and therefore has increased autonomy in its total programming. The funding change will take place over the next year, but will not adversely affect programming. Services will still be provided county-wide.

Statistics

Overall programming has continued to reach increasing numbers of Senior Citizens throughout the county. For the same six month period of time in 1977 and 1978, over 1700 more older persons were seen on the van, with the van making few stops and visiting slightly fewer sites. The program began with an average of 9.8 visitors per site, the first month, increased to 10.9 during July to December 1977, and further increased to 14.8 during July to December, 1978. Follow through with referrals made had more than doubled. Further, the number of revisits to the van during July to December 1978 increased by well over 50%. Continued increases along these same lines are fully expected.

Projections

The statistics indicate acceptance and use of the Sr. Citizens' Mobile Drop-In Center. A number of factors contribute to the program's success: visibility, good public relations by the consumers, coordination with other community agencies, staff enthusiasm, and the van's adaptability to program needs. However, as is always true with successful programs, increased utilization means increased demand for additional, needed services. These might include more off-site programs such as formal, time-limited group discussions at nutrition sites, senior clubs and senior housing units (nursing homes, boarding homes). Also, it is hoped that outreach, home visits to the homebound, isolated older persons becomes a more frequent occurrence.

In all the programs with which the Sr. Citizens Mobile Drop-In Center deals and plans for, the original conclusion reached by St. Clare's Mental Health Center in the planning stages for this service have been confirmed. Service groups have been identified and continue to dictate the priority of services offered. Program experience has shown that seniors are viable resources to a community, especially when their physical and emotional needs are no longer inhibiting their general functioning.

REFERENCES

1. Stuart, M. R. and K. J. Mackey, "Mobile Center Links Providers with Isolated Senior Citizens," *Hospitals, J.A.H.A.,* Vol. 52 (January 1, 1978), pp. 101–105.
2. Op. cit., p. 103.

PROMOTION

INTRODUCTION

The promotional area, more so than any of the other C.A.P.S., is mistaken most frequently to be the one and only area of health care marketing. In fact, the results of an informal survey of the meaning of the title of *Marketing Health Care* by Robin MacStravic (published by Aspen Systems Corporation in 1977) indicated that to health professionals it meant promoting or advertising health care, when in fact that was only a minor part of that book. Much literature in the health care field has focused on the ethics of marketing or advertising. For that reason, two readings on those concerns have been included, "Ethics Aspect of Advertising Debated" and "To Market, to Market, to Sell a Hospital."

Is it a gimmick or is it marketing? This is the question readers should be asking as they are exposed to increasingly less traditional methods of delivering health care. If the act (for example a steak, champagne, and candlelight dinner for the parents of a newborn the night before checkout) is done only for its short-term impact and not linked to longer term goals or a result of a change dictated by research, then that act is nothing more than a gimmick. If the act is a reaction (to get a higher maternity census) to a symptom (e.g., falling usage of an obstetrics ward), rather than a solution (reallocation of resources from the maternity ward to physical therapy) to a problem (population shift to elderly and declining birth rate), then it is a gimmick. Unfortunately, the examples in most of the literature are not complete enough for evaluation of more than the newsworthy flashy act.

Promotion in health care marketing goes beyond advertising to include personal selling, health education, public relations, incentives, and atmospherics. If the health care consumer is defined as the physician, as well as the patient, then the use of personal selling as a promotional technique for health care delivery is more obvious. The greatest difference between goods marketing and health care marketing exists in the remaining four areas. For example, the health education process is an important promotional function, especially in the development of preventive health care behavior. The third article, "Consumer Behavior and Health Care Change: The Role of Mass Media," explores the use of the media to bring about changes in such consumer behavior as smoking. Mass media have not been extremely successful, and this article looks at why.

A goods marketer would refer to any nonpaid form of advertising as publicity, and in many corporations this is a relatively small and obscure function. This is not true for health care. Public relations is a very important function and is emphasized heavily. Public relations or liaison efforts between the organization and the various publics is critical in building goodwill and support of the community as well as developing an understanding of how the organization works. The fourth article in this section, "Consumer Services: Inhospital Reachout," discusses the development of a consumer service representative and the results as an example of the liaison function of public relations.

The last two elements of promotion—incentives and atmospherics—while not the exclusive domain of health care marketing, nonetheless are important in the delivery of health care and consumer satisfaction. Incentives may be more valuable in the future in promoting preventive health care behavior. Atmospherics will gain in importance as consumer orientation becomes more predominant in health care delivery. The consumer's perception of the design and contents of the building or office may affect the way patients feel, thus contributing to their recovery. The article, "The Birth of a Service: Conceived by the Patient, Delivered by the Hospital," while found in the section on Service Development, discusses atmospherics as a part of the process of service development.

18. Ethics Aspect of Advertising Debated

CHRISTY MARSHALL

Reprinted from the April 1977 issue of *Modern Healthcare*, Copyright, Crain Communications, Inc. All rights reserved.

Recently in Washington, the American Hospital Association proposed guidelines on advertising to its board of trustees. The AHA proposal warned against comparative tactics, stating it is unethical to boast of being "more than, better than or newer than" any other hospital.

It also denounced the promotion of a single member of any hospital staff as a marketing tool for the hospital as a whole. The board postponed passage pending further revision.

Immediately the question arises—why would the AHA be concerned? Hospitals traditionally have scoffed at such commercial ploys. But not so anymore. Hospitals are increasingly marketing their services to patients and doctors. For example, Sunrise Hospital in Las Vegas is running a heavy TV, radio and print campaign promoting the hospital's special offer to win a first-class, all-expenses-paid Mediterranean cruise for two. The chance to win is open to anyone who checks into Sunrise on a Friday or Saturday. The hospital is spending approximately $10,000 a month backing its campaign. [See Exhibit 1.]

Mt. Sinai Hospital, Chicago, took out an eight-page insert in the January 13 regional issue of *Time*, giving the results of a Harris survey it recently had commissioned (*Modern Healthcare*, February 1977). The ad ran in lieu of the traditional annual report.

Skokie Valley Community Hospital, Skokie, IL, has been running a series of ads in Chicago newspapers on its alcoholic treatment unit. Two years ago, California hospitals fought the malpractice battle with a series of newspaper ads informing the public what the issue entailed. Some hospitals are including their own supplements in Sunday papers—Augustana Hospital in Chicago recently sent out 10,000 flyers to neighborhood residents informing them what their local hospital had to offer.

Dr. John McLaren, former internist, has been named vice-president for marketing at Evanston Hospital, the first of his kind. The appointment was made, Dr. McLaren said, "to help the hospital adopt a more aggressive marketing position," and to coordinate activities between Evanston and its second hospital, Glenbrook.

As the trend picks up momentum, one wonders why now? Philip Kotler, Northwestern University professor and acclaimed "granddaddy of nonprofit marketing," attributes it to the fact that "hospitals have gone to an overbedded position, forcing them to be more competitive."

The hospital directs its marketing at two different audiences—physicians and the community. To entice the medical staff, more and more hospitals are now providing what Prof. Kotler terms "ego services," such as saunas, tennis courts, chauffeur service and special hospital equipment. For the community, hospitals are trying to improve relations and promote their services—expecially their outpatient facilities.

Marketing has long been strong in proprietary hospital chains, yet is still revolutionary for its nonprofit brethren. And within those institutions, some traditionalists are objecting to the trend.

"Hospitals are not used to the idea of marketing," said Ted Tyson, director of the hospital department of Britt & Frerichs, Chicago, marketing consultant. "The word is unintelligible to them. They don't sell their services—they provide them."

Dr. McLaren found initial skepticism among his medical colleagues regarding his new post, too, but since then, those colleagues "have gotten quite in tune with marketing. All physicians are entrepreneurs. In a sense, they are marketing themselves."

Ireland Educational Corp. in Denver has been conducting marketing seminars for hospital administrators in cities across the country. The director, Richard Ireland, has found a strong interest in marketing by hospital administrators.

"But we avoid the image of marketing through advertising," Mr. Ireland said. "They aren't receptive to it; they don't understand advertising."

At Mount Sinai, the administration anticipated loud objections to their recent *Time* ad venture.

"The board of directors picked up the tab to allay any criticism," Mr. Ralston said. "You have a very sticky situation here. With the cost of hospital services so high, people complain: How can you spend so much money on advertising?"

Mr. Ralston contends advertising can be used to help the public in health education. "Hospitals should be doing institutional ads and they have to be ethical," he concluded.

According to Dwight Geduldig, manager of public affairs at the AHA (and according to the proposed AHA guidelines), hospital advertising should be a statement of fact of what the hospital provides. Also, the hospital can ethically make the public aware of unused services.

"As long as the intent is to better serve the public, we subscribe fully to hospitals advertising," commented Tom Drews, director of the Chicago Hospital Assn.

Jack Smith, of the California Hospital Assn., sees advertising as a means of "extending themselves [hospitals] into the community more rather than staying aloof. But you cannot lure people to your hospital."

With nonprofit hospitals' advertising still in its infancy, many people wonder how far it will grow.

Exhibit 1 Sunrise Hospital's Promotion Ad

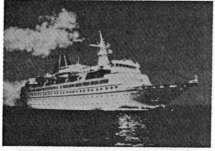

19. To Market, to Market, To Sell a Hospital

SUSAN NICHOLS

Reprinted from *Tennessee Hospital Times* by Susan Nichols, Assitant Director, Public Relations, Tennessee Hospital Association, by permission of the Tennessee Hospital Association, © Vol. 19, no. 1 (Jan. 1978).

"Should I advertise my hospital? If so, just what do I advertise and to whom should my advertisement be directed? Is it really the acceptable thing to do?"

Those are the questions that hundreds of hospital administrators are beginning to ask themselves and others. Although hospital advertising is not strictly a new concept, it seems that way due to its sudden proliferation. The Federal Trade Commission (FTC) has given cautious approval to hospital advertising. The American Hospital Association (AHA) has recently given us guidelines for advertising. The Federation of American Hospitals (FAH) has advocated the concept through their recent decision to approach the AHA and the American Medical Association about a jointly funded advertising project. Blue Cross and Blue Shield are currently in the second phase of a major advertising campaign and finally, a few brave and fairly innovative hospitals are actually buying ad space in newspapers, magazines and on television.

"So, if all these health care agencies say it's okay, why don't we go ahead and do it" you ask? We can't and don't intend to answer that question for you. All we can do is tell you about what's being done around the country and let you make the final determination.

AHA Guidelines

The long awaited *Guidelines on Advertising by Hospitals*, formulated for AHA by a committee of the American Society for Hospital Public Relations, was finally approved by the Board of Trustees and the House of Delegates of the AHA last August [1977] in Atlanta. Although some health care executives feel the guidelines are not specific and give no real help to the advertising dilemma, the guidelines do serve the purpose for which they were intended. It seems the guidelines arose amid controversy over some hospitals being more aggressive than others in using paid advertising for various communications purposes.

The guidelines neither recommend nor discourage paid or free advertising to further community awareness. Their aim is to provide

157

benchmarks for hospitals. According to AHA, at the basis of the guidelines is a concern that hospitals maintain their ethical sense of public accountability and that hospitals reflect fairness, honesty, accuracy and impartiality in their communications activities.

The guidelines declare five purposes for advertising. The first is advertising to educate the public about available hospital services. The hospital must assume. . . .responsibility for making services which may have an impact on the health of the. . . .community known. In addition, most health care facilities today find it desirable and economical to assure efficient utilization of expensive facilities by informing the public of those services through public relations or advertising.

The second purpose is to educate the public about health care. Hospitals are increasingly playing the role of public health educators. Advertising used to promote health classes or to describe good health practices is in the best interest of the community.

Accounting to the public is the third acceptable purpose for advertising. Hospitals have a moral and ethical responsibility to account to their community on a regular basis that their resources are being invested wisely. When this accountability cannot be accomplished effectively through other means, newspaper supplements, ads, tv and radio time are appropriate.

Advertising may also be used by the hospital to seek public support for funds or political assistance. But advertising to generate support for the hospital's point of view on legislative issues or political candidates can raise serious questions concerning the hospital's tax status and should be reviewed by legal counsel.

The final acceptable purpose for advertising is employment recruitment. Advertising for employment is legitimate, but must conform to honesty and legal requirements.

The AHA guidelines also list what can be considered acceptable content for hospital ads. The advertisement must be truthful, accurate and fair. Hospital advertising is an issue of such sensitivity that the truthfulness and accuracy of content must be beyond question. Self-aggrandizement of one hospital at the expense of another may be counterproductive and, if inaccurate could lead to charges of libel and claims for damage.

Quality comparisons, either direct or implied, between a hospital's services, facilities, or employees and those of another hospital may be counterproductive and libelous.

All advertising should be limited to statements of irrefutable fact. Claims of the "Best and Most Efficient" are always open to criticism and should be avoided. In addition, any institutional advertising that may directly or indirectly promote the professional practice of individuals within the hospital should be reviewed in light of possible embarrassment to the individuals or to possible violation of valid restriction of either ethical or statutory nature.

National AHA Campaign

With these guidelines firmly in hand, the AHA launched a major advertising campaign of their own. According to AHA President, Alex McMahon, the goal of the campaign is to put hospitals back into perspective for the American public. "We have undertaken this project for two reasons," McMahon said. "First, because the need for decision makers to understand the hospital industry has never been greater. Second, because we must remind the public of the hospital mission and what it represents. There is a tendency for public attention to focus on high costs without consideration of the services and care hospitals provide. This advertising campaign is an assertive and aggressive approach to reminding people of the good which hospitals do."

The cost of the AHA advertising campaign is $144,000. The budget was funded through AHA advertising revenues instead of from membership dues. The campaign consists of two levels. The first level consisted of ads, which have appeared in the *Wall Street Journal,* the *New York Times* and the *Washington Post*, that were aimed primarily at decision makers. The ads are a major commentary on the reasons for rising hospital costs. The second level of ads, . . . [run] in newspapers in 10 major metropolitan areas, stress the services hospitals provide their communities. They reinforce the idea that the public receives a highly valuable service for their hospital dollars.

In addition to buying advertising space in major newspapers, the AHA mailed the ads to all member institutions encouraging their use as educational materials, public service messages or paid advertising in local newspapers.

Although sufficient time has not passed to fully analyze public opinion toward the AHA ads, initial response has been fairly positive.

Blue Cross and Blue Shield Join Forces

The AHA move to advertising may seem like a progressive undertaking to some, but AHA is still well behind Blue Cross and Blue Shield in terms of budget and duration of advertising campaigns.

The Blues have been using paid advertising for years. It was only recently that they decided to combine their budgets and advertise as one entity. The first phase of their joint effort began in September 1976

Exhibit 1   Example of Ad Banned by the American Medical Association in 1947

**** 33

ADVERTISEMENT

STOMACH DISORDERS

Dropped Stomach, Ulcers and Chronic Ailments Dangerous If Not Correctly Diagnosed

Dr.   of This City, With Fluoroscopic X-Ray Learns True Cause of Your Troubles and Never Treats Unless He Knows

For over 25 years Dr. has successfully practiced here and in hospitals. His broad experience and fatherly advice is causing many relieved patients to advise others who suffered for years to take advantage of the valuable service he now gives in his private practice for fees within your power to pay.

Dr.   is now offering all who suffer a careful Full $5.00 Fluoroscopic

X-RAY   EXAMINATION

Including Urinalysis, Blood Pressure Tests and Physical Examination

For Only

$1.00

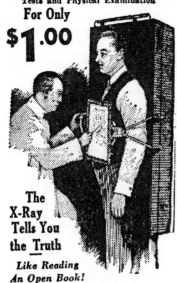

The X-Ray Tells You the Truth

Like Reading An Open Book!

If Stomach Is Dropped, Ulcers Present, Cause of Vomiting, Bloating, Gas, Pains, Fluttering Heart and Other Troubles are Revealed to You In This Complete Examination.

Through Diathermy and Other Modern Electrical Appliances and Correct Medical Treatment Used by Doctor Relief Is Often Given in Many Stubborn Cases in a Single Treatment.

He invites you to accept his liberal offer now, before your ailment is beyond help of even this modern, scientific treatment!

If You Suffer—Don't Wait!

Conditions such as Anemia, Asthma, Catarrh, Cystitis, Nerve Weakness, Diabetes, Neuralgia, Neuritis, Gout, Rheumatism, Toxemia, Insomnia, Liver and Kidney Trouble, Nose and Throat Troubles, Blood, Skin and many other disorders are successfully treated.

CONSULTATION CONFIDENTIAL

Clip and bring this coupon below. It entitles you to the complete $5.00 examination for only $1.00. No Waiting. Come NOW!

Dr.

BROADWAY, N. Y. C.
54th St. and B'way)
Hours: 9 A. M. to 7 P. M. Any Week Day
BRING THIS SPECIAL COUPON   M-94

and cost $2,306,000. The second phase began September 1977 and [ran] until June 1978 at a cost of $2,550,000.

The advertising is designed to stress hospital cost containment, more effective use of the health care system and better health habits on the part of citizens.

The Blue Cross and Blue Shield ads have appeared on major television networks, in popular magazines and in newspapers. From September to December of 1976, the Blues sponsored commercials 24 times on network news and sports telecasts.

According to Blue Cross officials, response to the ads has been "very little." However, they consider that a positive sign because they feel the public will usually respond to what they don't like.

FAH EFFORT

The Federation of American Hospitals recently hired a New York advertising firm to come up with a proposal for hospital advertising. The firm recommended that the most efficient use of ad time is on television and suggested a $1 million campaign lasting six months.

The FAH Board approved the concept and appropriated $100,000 toward its inception. The committee formed to handle the campaign was asked to approach the AMA and the AHA about a possible joint venture. Both organizations expressed serious reservations. The AHA had received less than favorable response from an earlier television ad campaign and the AMA was in the midst of a controversy with the Federal Trade Commission concerning physician advertising.

The gist of the proposed campaign was a series of ads aimed at consumers explaining the quality of health care. When we contacted Andrew Miller, President-Elect of FAH, he said that the organization would take the original program and develop it for use by individual member institutions. "We will support the advertising effort of our member hospitals," Miller said. "We'll try to thrust all of our advertising in the same direction and provide the staff and expertise to assist our members."

Hospitals Join the Act

Individual hospitals are also getting into the advertising act. Perhaps the most prominent and controversial advertising campaign by a hospital at this time is the one being used by Sunrise Hospital Medical Center in Las Vegas, Nevada. The hospital advertises a chance at a recuperative, all expense paid trip (up to $4000) anywhere

Exhibit 2 The American Hospital Association Used this Ad and Similar Ones in Several Metropolitan Newspapers Across the U.S. During a Recent Print Media Ad Campaign.

What's it worth to hear him say, "I'll be seeing you"

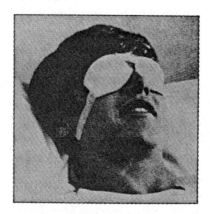

How about 70¢ a day? ... because that's all per capita hospital costs in America come to. That's about $255 a year. Less than what it costs a wage earner for Social Security taxes; less than one-third of his income taxes; and less than fuel and maintenance for the family car ... for the finest hospital care in the world.

Yet there are those who claim that hospital costs are too high, and should be "price controlled". We ask: too high compared to what? ...compared to when? To 1940? When the recovery rate from coronary occlusion was less than 50% -- compared to 85% today. To 1950? When survival from the first kidney transplants was "zero" -- compared to 80% today. Or to 1950, when average life expectancy was 68 years -- compared to 72.5 years today. And compared to price index increases since 1970, medical costs have risen less than food, fuel and utilities, and only slightly more than housing.

The fact is that aside from simple inflation and the ever-increasing cost of government regulation, the most significant factor in rising health-care cost has been improvements in care and treatment -- and a longer, healthier, fuller life for you and your family.

We think it's worth it ... to make hearts beat again, legs run again, eyes see again. For our profit-and-loss is measured in lives. And we think that's the way you want it.

Today's Hospital Care -- it's the bargain of your life.

in the world the patient chooses if the patient enters the hospital on a Friday or Saturday. The stated purpose of this offer is to foster better utilization of hospital services on the weekend.

Sunrise Hospital is a total health care facility and must have staff prepared for work seven days a week on a non-stop basis. As with most hospitals, surgical facilities are underutilized by physicians on the weekends. Sunrise wanted to encourage patients to enter on these days in an effort to better balance their workload and make greater use of available facilities. All of this, in turn, holds down the cost of care for the patient.

The advertising program began in 1976 with ads offering a 5.25 percent cash rebate to patients who entered the hospital on Friday or Saturday. Although community response to this program was overwhelming with a 30 to 50 percent increase in weekend admissions, Sunrise soon had to withdraw the offer. Large insurance companies began deducting the rebate for themselves and other companies began to boycott the hospital.

The rebate ad was soon followed by an offer of a recuperative Mediterranean Cruise for two which finally evolved into the offer of a trip anywhere in the world. (See the previous selection by Marshall in this book.)

Response to the ad has been good for the hospital. They have a year-round medical-surgical occupancy rate of 92 percent. The hospital has, in fact, received both a word of praise and one of caution from HEW Deputy Secretary for Health Planning and Evaluation, Dr. Karen Davis. Dr. Davis says that HEW is in favor of the ads if they result in a hospital running at peak efficiency seven days a week. However, if the ads extend the average length of stay, cause a rise in the hospital's annual number of admissions, or otherwise lead to unnecessary use of hospitals by patients who could be cared for just as well in less expensive surroundings, HEW is opposed to their use.

Another series of ads which were brought to our attention recently were sponsored by four hospitals in Long Beach, California. They appeared for a week in a local newspaper. The ads were designed to explain some of the reasons for rising hospital costs and remind the public of the quality medical care they are receiving for their health care dollar.

Prior to the ads appearing in the newspaper, the hospitals sent out a preview packet to health care leaders to alert them to the campaign. On the cover of the bright red packet were imprinted the words, "Warning: The U.S. Government Can Be Hazardous To Your Health."

These are just two of hundreds of examples of advertising by hospitals and the number is increasing daily. Many metropolitan and state hospital associations are establishing committees on marketing and advertising. Hospitals are frequently using Sunday newspaper supplements to explain their services, print progress reports and observe special occasions.

Big Brother is Watching

While all of this appears to be running smoothly and nobody has really goofed badly with their advertising schemes, you better believe big brother (alias Federal Trade Commission) is keeping an eagle eye aimed in our direction.

There are no canons or anything in writing that forbids hospitals from advertising such as the regulations for the practice of law or medicine. So far, all the FTC has said is that hospital advertising "must be truthful."

The Federal Trade Commission, however, is causing advertising headaches for the American Medical Association (AMA). Traditionally, the AMA has discouraged advertising by physicians for the purpose of solicitation of patients. The original ban on advertising was made in 1847 to avoid the type of blatant advertising which was associated with snake oil and other "miraculous cures."

In December of 1975, the Federal Trade Commission filed suit against the AMA charging that the Association's Principles of Medical Ethics prohibited doctors from generating business by advertising, price competition and competitive practices resulting in restraint of trade. On the other hand, the AMA says they are trying to protect the public from being defrauded by outrageous claims made by opportunists. Furthermore, the AMA has said that they encourage doctors to advertise their office hours, locations and specialties.

The case is currently in court and the final decision may eventually have an impact on hospital advertising.

The American Hospital Association says that about 10 percent of the 7,000 American hospitals have taken out display advertisements. So far, the ads have been acceptable. However, as more of us get in the act, will ads become highly competitive and gimmicky? Time will tell.

Currently the Tennessee Hospital Association has no definitive stand on hospital advertising. THA has neither accepted or rejected the AHA guidelines on advertising. THA would, however, suggest caution and moderation in advertising. The science of marketing health care is relatively new. We will keep you informed as developments arise.

Exhibit 3 This Ad Is One of a Series Developed by Four Hospitals in Long Beach, California. The Series Ran for One Week in a Local Newspaper.

WHEN GOVERNMENT RATIONS HEALTH CARE, WHERE WILL YOU BE IN LINE?

When the Arabs withheld oil, we all lined up at the pumps.

When the U.S. government' rations health care, how will you like lining up at the hospital?

Americans pay nine cents on the dollar for all health care expenses — doctors, hospitals, medicine. But the U.S. government says we're spending too much.

What has that nine cents helped you to buy?

Added years of health and life — 20 years more than our parents could expect.

New sight for the 65 year old with cataracts.

The ability to walk again for the 24 year old accident victim.

Life saving heart surgery for the 45 year old.

Nine cents is a drop in the bucket compared to the huge sums government spends on foreign aid, military forces,

highways, bureaucratic paper shuffling.

But the government says they've got to cut someplace. And that someplace is your health.

You cut costs. You cut quality. And then who gets what and how much?

It means rationing the amount of health, of added years of life, that you get.

Your locally elected officials are working to protect your freedom and your rights. They need to know what you think. Let them hear from you.

We've been working for nearly three quarters of a century to provide you with the best health care in the world.

Let us know what you think.

Write: "Four Hospitals"
P.O. Box 2860
Long Beach, CA 90801

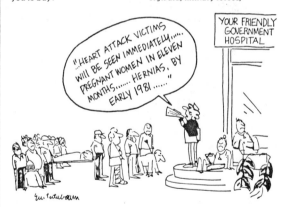

Together We Can Do Something About It

Endorsed by the Long Beach Area Chamber of Commerce

Long Beach Community Hospital
Memorial Hospital Medical Center of Long Beach
Pacific Hospital of Long Beach
St. Mary Medical Center — Bauer Hospital

20. Consumer Behavior and Health Care Change: The Role of Mass Media

THOMAS S. ROBERTSON AND
LAWRENCE H. WORTZEL

Reprinted with permission from *Advances in Consumer Research*, Vol. 4, 1977, pp. 525–527.

ABSTRACT

Mass media have considerable potential for affecting health behavior. The pervasiveness of mass media and the exposure levels of broad segments of society suggest that mass media may be an important *information source* regarding health and a relevant *socialization force* regarding health attitudes and behavior. Nevertheless, research evidence indicates that most mass media campaigns oriented toward changing health care habits fail. The objectives of this paper are to analyze *why* health care campaigns fail and to derive generalizations for more effective use of mass media by health care professionals.

OVERVIEW

The role of mass media in affecting knowledge, attitudes, and behavior toward health care may be thought of in terms of the following two dimensions.

1. Mass media may impact health knowledge, attitudes and behavior both in a *deliberate* sense through "campaigns" that are specifically designed for such impact, and in an *unintended* or "incidental learning" sense through material that contains health-related information, but which is not specifically intended to impact health knowledge, attitudes or behavior.
2. In both cases, mass media may act either as a "change agent" or as a "reinforcing agent"—that is, media may function in such a way as to *change* knowledge, attitudes and behavior or to *confirm* existing behavior patterns. In these respects, the role of mass media in affecting health care is similar to their role in affecting knowledge, attitudes and behavior toward other products and services.

167

CAMPAIGN VERSUS UNINTENDED EFFECTS

Mass media *campaigns* are intended to communicate certain health care information with a view toward change in health habits. Examples include anti-smoking, seat belt usage, lower cholesterol, and hypertension identification campaigns.

Mass media may also have unintended effects in the sense that the average viewer is exposed to a regular diet of "medical" shows on television and also to large numbers of commercials for proprietary medicines. The learning from such programming and commercials may be in the form of "misinformation" and may not be compatible with good health habits. A national study by the Louis Harris Organization (1973), for example, concluded that mass media were second only to the individual's physician as a source of health information. Furthermore, much of the health information absorbed from television is likely to be under low involvement conditions and, therefore, processed without evaluation.

A logical question then is whether mass media depict an accurate profile of health, illness, and the value of medical services, drug products, or medical treatment. Some social critics suggest that mass media depict a distorted and stereotyped view of these topics with consequences for people's health beliefs, attitudes and behavior and for their probabilities of accessing the medical system under specified conditions. For example, to what extent does advertising for proprietary drugs convince people to search for simplistic solutions to medical symptoms that may be indicative of more serious problems? To what extent does cigarette advertising help people to deny or sublimate the medically dangerous effects of smoking?

The extent to which mass media either positively or negatively impact health is an important empirical question requiring systematic evidence to resolve. One study of television programming found that 30% of the health-related information was "useful" while the remaining 70% was inaccurate or misleading or both (Smith, 1972). This may suggest the magnitude of the potential problem, although this study is only one isolated piece of research evidence. Another study by Frazier et al. (1974) of dental health advertisements concluded that 43% of the information is inaccurate, misleading, or fallacious. The hypothesis may well be that mass media act more to misinform than to educate people about health and appropriate health habits.

CHANGE AGENT OR REINFORCING AGENT

The potential of mass media communications in the health care arena is generally phrased in terms of their promise for *changing* habits and life styles. However, the history of communication research indicates that the most persistent finding is that mass media act mainly to *reinforce* existing attitudes and behavior.

The ability of mass media to effect change is actually a function of a number of factors and requires certain conditions which we will develop later in this paper. Basically, however, the probability of *change* tends to be a function of how much commitment people have to existing behavior patterns. Under high commitment conditions, as is frequently the case in health care, bringing about change may indeed be a difficult undertaking. This is likely to be the case since health behavior is frequently rooted both in long term reinforcement patterns and in support by the individual's social environment. (In some special cases physical and psychological addiction patterns may also be a factor with which to contend.) A look at the evidence on health care campaigns supports the statement that most health care campaigns do not succeed among large numbers of intended subjects. The literature is replete with discouraging case studies.

Obesity. In summarizing the evidence on obesity, Stunkard (1975) sets forth five propositions: (1) most obese people do not enter treatment, (2) of those who do, most drop-out, (3) of those who remain, most do not lose much weight, (4) of those who lose weight most will regain it, and (5) many of those entering treatment pay a high emotional price. Nevertheless, Stunkard registers considerable hope based on behavior modification programs, which recently have improved the treatment of obesity. He implicitly rejects mass media as an important force in changing behavior.

Smoking. Anti-smoking campaigns have had limited success, at best. Cigarette consumption has not declined, despite communication campaigns and public policy initiatives protecting non-smokers. In fact, it is increasing among teenagers, especially among girls. However, there has been a change toward consumption of lower tar and nicotine cigarettes. Perhaps the consequence of messages about lower tar and nicotine cigarettes has been to convince smokers that smoking is becoming safer.

On the other hand, one potentially successful anti-smoking campaign was initiated, when counter-advertising messages were shown on television under the equal time provision of the Federal Communications Commission. Possibly the combination of smoking and counter-smoking commercials presented together acted similarly to a two-sided communication; however, it is unlikely that mass media counter-advertising alone accomplished the job.

Seat Belts. In a review of research on seat belt usage campaigns, Leon Robertson et al. (1974) report a general lack of positive results. These authors then initiated a well-controlled experimental study using split-cable television whereby one audience received messages advocating seat belt use and a matched audience on the other half of the cable did not receive messages. After a nine month period tracking actual seat belt usage behavior, the authors could only conclude that: "The campaign had no measured effect whatsoever on safety belt use" (p. 1077).

Community Fluoridation Programs. Despite endorsement by the United States Public Health Service and the Surgeon General, controlled fluoridation of community water supplies has more often been rejected than accepted by voters. Between 1950 and 1969, 1139 communities voted on fluoridation; the issue lost in 666 communities and won in 473 (HEW, 1970). One part of the difficulty is the complexity of the fluoridation issue and another part is voters' susceptibility to the fear appeals used by opponents.

Health Maintenance Organizations. Despite the advantages claimed for the HMO concept, enrollment campaigns have met with limited success—with a few notable exceptions (primarily the Kaiser plan). Perhaps the HMO concept is not as desirable as its advocates claim (Glasgow, 1972) or perhaps the benefits to consumers are not readily apparent and communication campaigns have underestimated the difficulties of changing medical behavior patterns.

Heart Disease. The most encouraging results on a mass media campaign are from the Stanford study conducting a program to reduce susceptibility to heart disease among residents of three communities. Instructional programs used in conjunction with mass media have documented attitudinal and behavioral changes in diet and cigarette smoking. The role of mass media alone in one community on a delayed continuity basis is almost as effective as the personal instruction-mass media combination (Maccoby and Farquhar, 1975). The cost-effectiveness of this campaign, however, is very much in question.

WHY HEALTH CAMPAIGNS FAIL, AND HOW TO HELP THEM SUCCEED

Analysis of the foregoing and other campaigns indicates that there are some basic reasons why most health care campaigns fail. These reasons may be summarized as follows:

1. Most health care campaigns operate without explicit objectives or with inappropriate or unrealistic objectives, probably because they are based on an inadequate understanding of the way mass communications work, and on an inadequate understanding of the marketing requirements of the "product" being promoted.
2. Most health care campaigns are non-programmatic; they are short-run, one-time efforts, while the behavior change they are designed to induce must continue in the long run.
3. The beneficial effects of the recommended behavior change are not immediately apparent to the consumer, and perhaps never will be.
4. Most health care campaigns fail to identify market segments within the total audience who require different communication approaches in line with their specific needs.

Setting Objectives and Assigning a Role to the Mass Media

It is not sufficient to seek knowledge change or attitude change without a mechanism for also achieving behavior change and it is difficult for the mass media to achieve behavior change. For example: most smokers have *knowledge* of the ill effects of smoking and may have a negative *attitude* toward smoking. Therefore, presenting them with more knowledge as to the negative effects of smoking is unlikely to have much impact. Instead, a communication campaign must be linked to a behavior change mechanism other than mass communications (such as behavior modification group enrollment) if the campaign is to be successful. But behavior change even so induced is unlikely to persist in the long run unless its beneficial effects are continuously reinforced, since the beneficial results from the behavior change are not apparent in the short run and since there may also be some gratifications attached to the previous behavior.

Although non-smoking is a regularly repurchased "product," this is a different marketing situation from the usual consumer packaged goods situation in which advertising is used to achieve trial, and in which reinforcement from use of the product is a significant force in accomplishing continuing use of the product. An important function of mass communications in changing health behavior must be to *reinforce* new behavior, since use of the "product" is insufficient reinforcement in itself. Fortunately, this is a role which mass media have continually demonstrated an ability to perform well. Nevertheless, behavior change must be accomplished first, and by means other than mass media.

As we have noted, most health campaigns are short-run, start and stop efforts, with little long-term systematic and programmatic planning. Yet, changing health is likely to involve both multiple channels of persuasion and regular long term reinforcement. In summary, people must be moved through a decision sequence which is likely to take some significant amount of time and different means of persuasion [that] may have complementary and cumulative impact, and may be necessary to achieve persistent behavior change.

Segmentation

Most health care campaigns try to reach everyone. Yet, not all segments of the market are as likely to change and different segments may require different incentives for change. It is incumbent on the change agent to specify the market segments likely to be receptive to change and to expect that different messages focused on different needs may be effective with different demographic and psychographic segments.

Examination of needs by segment may be mandatory. For example: smoking provides gratification for smokers; it fulfills certain needs. These needs may relate to anxiety patterns or may be tied to social interaction patterns (Wortzel and Clarke, 1977). Programs to help reduce smoking, we might argue, should help find alternatives for the continued satisfaction of these needs. Basically, if we are to change health we must do so in line with people's needs. It does little good to scare people, insult people, etc., except under certain extreme conditions. Changed health patterns must be shown to be in line with the audience's self-perceived needs.

Segmentation is also critical if mass media are used to support a campaign in which behavior change has been accomplished by other means. Reaching the yet unchanged will be wasteful, if not counterproductive in light of possible future efforts. It is essential to reach the changed in order to reinforce the behavior changing mechanism.

CONCLUSION: PRINCIPLES FOR HEALTH CARE CHANGE

Following is a set of tentative propositions for the successful design and implementation of health care campaigns.

1. Mass media communication by itself may be effective in initiating change, but generally only if the change sought is minor

and consumers have low information needs. This is seldom the case in health care.

2. Mass media communication will generally be most effective at an early point in the health decision change process whereas personal sources will generally be most effective later in the decision change process.

   a. Mass media communication objectives, therefore, must be tied toward encouraging people to access the professional health care system, or to sensitize them to other sources of communication.

   b. The peer and professional system will constitute the subsequent supporting mechanism necessary to bring about actual change.

3. It is the cumulative effect of a communication campaign that eventually results in behavior change.

   a. This indicates the need for repetition and reinforcement over time. Reinforcement of health change is a particularly important role for mass media.

   b. This indicates the need for multiple information sources which play complementary roles—including advertising, personal selling, peer support, and professional intervention.

4. Peer sources (personal influence) will be a particularly important source of legitimation and "reality testing" when the benefits of change are not obvious or cannot be demonstrated in the short run. This is likely to be the case in much of health care.

5. Communication campaigns for health care—even when they make use of donated public media time and space—are not free. The real cost is the opportunity cost if the communication campaign could have been more successful.

6. A health care communication campaign must explicitly recognize the problem of selective perception—that those who see the message may be those who are already concerned about the issue and engaging in recommended change activities.

7. A communication campaign may have to provide support for change within a family or peer group context. Obesity, for example, may be tied to family diet habits and change may depend on family involvement.

8. Communication messages must be keyed to the needs of the market segment being reached. It is necessary to offer positive alternatives and not simply to denigrate the individual's existing health habits.

9. Low returns should be expected in a communication campaign. Most advertising and persuasion seeks small levels of change—in the range of 3 to 5 percent of the audience per year. Mass conversion in the short-run is indeed a rare phenomenon.

REFERENCES

Frazier, P. Jean, Joanna Jenny, Ron Ostman and Charles Frenick, "Quality of Information in Mass Media: A Barrier to the Dental Health Education of the Public," *Journal of Public Health Dentistry*, Vol. 34, Fall, 1974, pp. 244–257.

Glasgow, John M. "Prepaid Group Practice as a National Health Policy: Problems and Perspectives," *Inquiry*, Vol. 9, September 1972, pp. 3–15.

Harris, Louis Organization, A study cited in *The Report of the President's Committee on Health Education*, New York, 1973.

HEW, *Fluoridation Census 1969* (Bethesda, Md: U.S. Dept of HEW, 1970).

Maccoby, Nathan and John W. Farquhar, "Bringing the California Health Report Up to Date," *Journal of Communication*, Vol. 26, Winter, 1976, pp. 56–67.

Maccoby, Nathan and John W. Farquhar, "Communication for Health: Unselling Heart Disease," *Journal of Communication*, Vol. 25, Summer, 1975, pp. 114–126.

Robertson, Leon S., Albert B. Kelley, Brian O'Neill, Charles W. Wixom, Richard S. Eiswirth and William Haddon, "A Controlled Study of the Effect of Television Messages on Safety Belt Use," *American Journal of Public Health*, Vol. 64, November, 1974, pp. 1071–1080.

Smith, Frank A., Goeffrey Trivaz, David A. Zuehlke, Paul Lowinger and Thieu L. Nghiem, "Health Information During a Week of Television," *New England Journal of Medicine*, Vol. 286, March 2, 1972, pp. 516–520.

Stunkard, Albert J., "Presidential Address-1974: From Explanation to Action in Psychosomatic Medicine: The Case of Obesity: *Psychosomatic Medicine*, Vol. 37, May-June 1975, pp. 195–236.

Wortzel, Lawrence H. and Roberta Clarke. "Environmental Protection for the Non-Smoker: Consumer Behavior Aspects of Encouraging Non-Smoking," *Advances in Consumer Research*, Vol. V, Association for Consumer Research, 1978.

21. Consumer Services: Inhospital Reachout

MARSHALL P. GAVIN

Reprinted, with permission, from *Hospitals, Journal of the American Hospital Association*, Vol. 49, no. 14, July 16, 1975, pp. 65–67. Copyright 1975, American Hospital Association.

Psychologist Erich Fromm defined alienation as "a mode of experience in which the person experiences himself as an alien."[1] Such an individual feels unable to control his own destiny. His existence seems to be a product of outside forces that are too large, too complex, and too remote for him to influence—big business, big labor, and big government. Which of us has not felt first the frustration, then the rage, and finally the humiliation of having our individuality ignored when attempting to correspond with a computerized billing system or trying to convince a Directory Assistance telephone operator to give us a street address as well as the party's phone number? How often today do we experience the personal relationships and mutual trust that were commonplace between individuals and their local merchants years ago?

Fromm suggests that when individuals are alienated from personal relationships through which they had been able to influence conditions that affect them adversely, "they manifest themselves in the sphere of the public realm." In other words, feeling powerless to change those forces upon which they see themselves as being totally dependent, the alienated abdicate responsibility and expediently turn to "all-powerful" big government to make conditions better in their behalf. Experience has shown us that this behavior is typical of the alienated personality frequently observed among consumer activists, who are quick to seek government sanctions and controls rather than risk further humiliation by personally attempting to influence the establishment.

If we are correct in our premise that consumer activism is an attempt to overcome feelings of helplessness and loss of personal worth that result from the alienating forces in our culture, we should expect the underlying motivations of the consumer movement to be an attempt to remove the causes of alienation and anxiety. Specifically, we should expect the basic motivation of the consumer movement to be the protection and enhancement of the individual's identity and the attainment of consumer influence over conditions and events that affect him. Supporting our premise, the Consumer's Bill of Rights, advanced in

175

1963 in the First Report of President Kennedy's Consumer Advisory Council, sought protection and influence for the individual: "the rights of safety, to be informed, to choose, and to be heard."

Reflecting upon this bill of rights, let us ask ourselves, Does the hospital patient feel safe, fully informed, able to choose, and capable of being heard and of influencing the events that affect him? The hospital environment denies the individual those values that are at the very basis of the consumer movement. We would suggest that even complaints over hospital charges and patients' bills are usually not money issues, but rather quality of life issues. After all, 84.2 percent of hospital costs are paid by third-party payers, not by the patients.[2] We believe that the patient and his family, feeling like aliens in this complex and impersonal environment over which they have little or no influence, are motivated by their anxiety to assert their own identities. In effect they are saying, "For all the money it cost for me to be here, why was I not treated more considerately, with more dignity?" [3] Assuming they receive satisfactory medical treatment, hospital patients and their families do not really want lower costs; they want more care.

A consumer services department was created at St. Anne's Hospital, Chicago, to counter the alienating forces inherent in a hospital environment. The new department was developed at no additional cost by combining the security department and the information center budgets. Its purpose is to clearly communicate our interest and concern for the patient and his family by actively reaching out, on a one-to-one basis, to provide a wide range of personal assistance. The philosophy and the slogan of the department is, "We wish you well." Where there had been the forbidding and hostile image of a policeman guarding a post, there is now the attractive, friendly, and helpful manager who is responsible for assisting patients and visitors in a given area with their problems. Where there had been threatening and sometimes violence-provoking police uniforms, there are now attractively coordinated red and blue sportswear outfits.[4,5] The former security department had been staffed mostly with retired policemen and night watchmen. The new department is staffed with bright, articulate, and enthusiastic men and women (CSRs), most of whom hold college degrees in the behavioral sciences.

One of the functions of the CSRs is to ensure the right of safety to life and property in an alert, courteous, and helpful manner similar to that of airline personnel, who must maintain strict security while providing friendly assistance to passengers. Rather than assuming that a visitor who wanders into a restricted area of the hospital has some malicious intent, the CSRs remain alert to possible undesirable intentions but treat such a person as lost or misdirected and escort him to the location he is seeking.

However, to prepare CSRs for any eventuality, they are thoroughly trained in modern and sophisticated security techniques. All CSRs must complete an intensive 30-hour course at the United States School of Law Enforcement in addition to their formal inservice education in human relations. This law enforcement training includes 25 hours of theory in protection, investigation, and law and five hours of practical training in the proper use of a weapon. Although all CSRs have been thoroughly trained in the use of a weapon and have been certified as law enforcement officers by the State of Illinois, they do not carry weapons but call on the municipal police department to deal with any circumstances in which the use of force may be necessary.

The consumer services department also addresses itself to the right of patients and visitors to be informed. The CSRs reassure patients who are waiting to be admitted and frankly explain the reasons for any delays, assist persons accompanying emergency patients in quickly learning the condition of the patients, and make referrals to the social services department when counseling or interagency coordination appears necessary. CSRs also distribute hospital brochures and other materials that are intended to help orient patients and visitors to the hospital's facilities and services. When a question arises for which a CSR does not have a ready answer, such as a question about insurance coverage or about the results of a laboratory test, the CSR arranges for the patient or visitor to speak to the person responsible for the information.

CSRs serve as ombudsmen on behalf of patients and visitors to help ensure their right to choose. If a patient's relative wishes to stay overnight to remain by the patient's side, the consumer services department will ensure that no bureaucratic policy will prevent the relative from making that choice. CSRs provide essential one-to-one relationships with patients and visitors and encourage them to make their preferences known, so that the consumer services department can work through the hospital organization to intervene on their behalf with the individuals responsible for the desired services. Such patient representation is crucial, because it also ensures patients' and visitors' right to be heard, to influence, and to reinforce their identities as individuals who can exert some control over the events that affect them.

RESULTS, BENEFITS

The establishment of the consumer services department has been surprisingly well received and well supported by hospital staff members whose duties made it difficult for them to deal with many patients' questions and nonmedical requests. Rather than feeling threatened by the CSRs' functioning as patient representatives, nurses have been enthusiastically referring patient food complaints, maintenance requests, and television rental follow-up to the consumer services department and have been enlisting the help of CSRs to interpret for non-English-speaking patients and visitors and even to reconcile family squabbles.

One of the important benefits of the consumer services department is that it seems to act as a catalyst for increasing the hospital staff's awareness that patients are not products but persons. Caring for patients seems to be growing. As a means of reducing consumer conflicts and generally improving community relations, a consumer services department is highly visible, inexpensive, and effective.

REFERENCES

1. Fromm, E. *The Sane Society*. New York: Holt, Rinehart, and Winston, Inc., 1955.

2. Consumer Advisory Council, *First Report*. Washington DC: U.S. Government Printing Office, Oct. 1963, p. 8.

3. Feldstein, S. The Rising Cost of Hospital Care. Washington, DC: Information Resources Press, 1971, p. 14.

4. Formula for Security. Part 1, *Hosp. Admin. Currents*. 18:4, June 1974.

5. Bradford, R. "Thief tells what to do to keep him out," *Mod. Hosp.* 121:87, July 1973.

SERVICE
DEVELOPMENT

INTRODUCTION

The last of the health care marketing C.A.P.S. is service development. The process of service development is one area where the concept of goods marketing can make a major contribution to the delivery of health care. The method by which a health care service is added now can be described best as a reaction. An example is a crisis situation in which the demand is so great that it forces the long-overdue development of a service to quell the discontent: a few medical specialists feel it would be a good idea to have a particular service, and the administrator reacts by providing the service to satisfy the specialists; the government dictates the service; or the competition just acquired a CAT scan so the board feels it also must get one to meet competition to keep up its technological image.

It is essential that particular attention be paid to the use of the word "process" of service development. A reaction is not planned, and certainly is not a process. The planning component of health care marketing is important and its effect is felt in the service development area as well as in the previous three areas (consideration, accessibility, promotion). The first article, "A Suggested Process for the Development of New Health Services," was selected because it offers the elements of a process to develop services that has been refined by the goods marketer and altered to fit the needs and constraints of service development in the health care industry.

The next article, "The Birth of a Service: Conceived by the Patient, Delivered by the Hospital," is an original manuscript based on the development process of "home style" childbirth service. While it does not illustrate all the elements of the process described in the previous article, some of those factors are present (for example, the inclusion of the patient along with the professionals to determine the nature and the scope of the service to be developed). Again, as in the three other areas, the accent on consumer orientation is the key to the marketing approach. An area yet to be explored is the antithesis of service development. A process of service elimination is needed. This process undoubtedly will be developed as the discipline of health care marketing matures.

The elements of the health care marketing C.A.P.S.: Consideration, Access or Availability, Promotion, and Service Development, compose what is referred to as the health care marketing mix. Each element must be part of an overall plan. What is done in one area affects all the others. Therefore, it is important to integrate each of the four areas with the others. The last two readings accomplish this goal. Marketing research provides the fuel for integration of the C.A.P.S. and the marketing plan provides the glue to hold them together.

22. A Process for Developing New Health Services

TONY BUSHMAN AND PHILIP COOPER

Reprinted with permission from *Health Care Management Review*, Winter 1980, pp. 41-48.

INTRODUCTION

By the early 1970s the time spent on the production of services was greater than the time spent on production of both durable and nondurable goods.[1] One of the most difficult areas for new market development is the service area. Since many services are intangible and thus difficult to fully and accurately communicate, it is difficult to develop and test them. While specific information about the failure rate of new services is scarce, new product failure rates may be an indication of new service failures. Failure rates have been recorded as low as 33 percent[2] to as high as 80 percent[3] or 89 percent.[4] These discrepancies arise from the use of different samples, different product categories and different definitions of failure. The important point is that all studies agree that failure is commonplace and substantial. If new service failure is only one-half that of new product failure, it is still something to be concerned about.

This article focuses on health services as an example for illustrating a procedural model for developing new services and reducing failure.

SUGGESTED NEW SERVICE PLANNING PROCEDURE

The procedure described here is a generalized set of steps for developing new health care services. This procedure is an ideal set of steps which should be adjusted to fit the characteristics of each organization and each proposed new service.

Health care service development has been chosen to focus on because of the increasing importance of the health care sector, (it currently accounts for about 10 percent of the GNP) and the current stress on cost containment. The use of a process is not a common practice. Such a process may minimize costs by avoiding the development of unwanted, underutilized or duplicate services. Figure 1 presents an overview of an eleven step process for the development of new health care services.

Figure 1 An Overview of the Eleven-Step Procedure

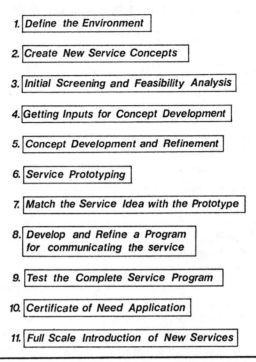

1. Define the Environment

2. Create New Service Concepts

3. Initial Screening and Feasibility Analysis

4. Getting Inputs for Concept Development

5. Concept Development and Refinement

6. Service Prototyping

7. Match the Service Idea with the Prototype

8. Develop and Refine a Program for communicating the service

9. Test the Complete Service Program

10. Certificate of Need Application

11. Full Scale Introduction of New Services

It should be pointed out that the steps are not necessarily hierarchical. The nature of the service under consideration or the organization may preclude the use of some of the steps or may dictate a different order.

Step One: Define the Environment

As one engages in the planning discipline, it is necessary to understand the boundaries of planning the system. Health care planners must work within the constraints of their environment and must know the needs of the environment as well as the mission and goals of the organization.

The health care industry is plagued by a series of constraints that make the development of new services difficult and challenging. Some of the major constraints include (for both profit and not-for-profit organizations): obtaining the approval of planning agencies (Health Systems Agencies); the education of several internal publics (e.g., staff, physicians, trustees) as to the availability, function, and operation of the service; the education of several external publics (such as referring physicians, patients, concerned public agencies) and working through the details of third party reimbursement.

An analysis of the environment should include an assessment of services already offered and a determination of how well the needs of internal and external publics are being met. This assessment should include a thorough review of the HSA Health Systems Plan to the point where the planner knows the complete plan.

Step Two: Create New Service Concepts (or finding new opportunities)

In the process of defining the environment, it is likely that new service needs will be identified. To increase the chance of defining new services that will be accepted by patients, doctors and staff, it is vital their opinions be sought and reflected in the definition of the new service. It is important that the health service administrator develop sensitivities to the external and internal environment in order to know what needs are not being met and when to seek changes. This requires frequent contact with the internal and external potential participants who are involved with the health service. Frequent communications and sensitivity to the environment will enhance the possibility of creating new services as a regular occurrence. However, new services can be more methodically developed through formal procedures. A number of useful service ideas are presented in Exhibit 1 and described below.

Exhibit 1 Examples of Useful Techniques to Generate New Service
Ideas

> 1. Role Playing
> 2. Internal Suggestions and Inducements
> 3. Brainstorming
> 4. Reverse Brainstorming
> 5. Benefit Checklist Technique
> 6. Free Association
> 7. Forced Association

1. Role Playing. This method requires the planner to place himself in the position of the potential user of the service. It is most often used early in the creative process or where time and funds are limited.

An example of how this can be done is described by Byrne.[5] While this example deals with the design of a physical facility for health care not a service, it demonstrated one way a designer gains insight to the needs of the eventual users. The process was to have doctors, nurses, patients and staff literally "walk through" a mockup and a hospital floor design that was laid on a large high school fieldhouse floor. The result was to uncover traffic patterns, check on door widths, determine comfortable waiting areas, etc., before the final design was established.

Another example of role playing is planners playing the role of an elderly person who is insecure and easily confused about hospital procedure. Here, the hospital could establish a consumer service representative to assist the elderly person.

Another problem may be that a patient does not really understand what the doctor has asked them to do after seeing the doctor. Role playing could lead to new services to avoid this problem.

2. **Internal Suggestions and Inducements.** The staff of the service center is eager to recommend improvements. Cash bonuses, performance awards or other rewards can be given to those who generate valuable ideas. This has been a useful approach in the manufacturing sector via the Scanlon Plan and suggestion boxes.[6]

A substantial advantage of this process is often overlooked in that suggestions which come from employees often have a built-in acceptance. Those who have generated the idea or those who realize that its origin was from within, will tend to support it and have high motivation to implement the idea.

3. **Brainstorming.** This method of creating new services is an uninhibited, rapid fire approach where ideas are offered without worrying about their merits.[7] The technique seeks large numbers of ideas through free wheeling thinking and withholds negative comments until after the pool of ideas has been exhausted.

After the ideas have been expressed, a brief assessment is made. Some ideas are combined with others and some are discarded because of infeasibility. Others are refined and developed further.

4. **Reverse Brainstorming.** This is often done as a prelude to the brainstorm sessions and encourages critical comments. The process basically involves listing all the things wrong with present health services and then goes through each negative feature one by one to determine ways of overcoming each problem.

5. **Benefit Checklist Technique.** This process involves listing benefits that health care consumers desire (see in Exhibit 2 below). In column B between any elements of the two lists, a third column (C) of new services can be created. For example, in Exhibit 2 below, the forced association of "speed" with "paramedics" stimulated the creation of an in-home preparation for heart failure. The other dotted lines shown in Exhibit 2 indicate other possible associations.

6. **Free Association.** This method of stimulating creativity must be used with care in order to identify new service opportunities. It is easy to stray into side issues with this technique. The first step is to write down a list of key problems or needs related to the health care service under consideration. For each key problem or need write down the idea suggested by the first problem or need. Exhibit 3 may help make this approach more understandable.

Reviewing the attributes of a new service that are associated with the key problems or needs, a new service labeled Consumer Service Representative might be developed.[8]

Exhibit 2 Example of Association Between Lists

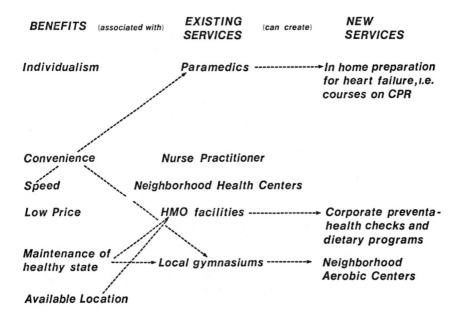

Exhibit 3 An Example of the Free Association of Attributes with Key
Problems or Needs

First Set of Key Problems/Needs	Associated Attributes of a New Service
Ignorance of Medicine or Hospital	Education of Patient
Delay of Entry into System	In-House coordination
Fear	Coping or stress exercises

7. **Forced Association.** This approach to creating new services is
a variation of the free association method. Key elements of a
situation are identified and then associated with each other in
various combinations. The various combinations are analyzed
and refined to define a new service. Exhibit 4 presents an application of a simplified situation.

While there are other techniques for creating new service ideas, the
preceding seven represent some of the most useful. Once a large
number of ideas has been generated, they must be evaluated and put
into a priority for development.

Step Three: Initial Screening and Feasibility Analysis

Formalized creativity sessions usually produce scores of ideas. Many
of the ideas will have serious debilitating problems which must be
assessed. A screening system must be developed which will accept the
good ideas and reject the bad ones. The most common mechanism for
assessing ideas is the screening committee.

The composition of the screening committee is very important. Its
members should have different backgrounds and have demonstrated a
good understanding of the needs which health service users have. For
example, a committee made up of a consumer, a representative of administration, a representative of the housekeeping department, a
nurse supervisor, and a staff physician has a mix of perspectives that
would cover many areas of concern in a hospital.

While it is possible for screening committees to arrive at collective
judgments by informal discussion and consensus, it is recommended
that most ideas be formally evaluated against an agreed upon list of
criteria. In most cases, the criteria can be given importance weightings
that can be used to construct relative success indices. Some of the most

Exhibit 4 Key Elements of a Health Delivery Center

Second set of Key Elements

		Safe / Accurate	*Accessible*
First set of Key Elements	*Automatic*	**New Service 1** *24 hour Credit Admissions Service*	**New Service 2** *Coin operated blood pressure machines*
	Safe / Accurate	——————	**New Service 3** *Nurse practitioner supervised center screening centers in shopping centers*

important criteria to include for assessment are judgments related to financial feasibility and serviceability from the viewpoint of whether the service technology is advanced enough to offer the service.

Step Four: Getting Further Inputs for Concept Development

Early in the development of a service idea, it is desirable to get inputs from potential users and those who might provide the service. This has a number of salutory effects that:

a. Improves the chances of creating an important, understand-able, relevant and usable service idea or concept.
b. Prepares the relevant parties for the future time when the serv-ice concept will become a real service.
c. Gives the parties a chance to register their pet peeves, and to feel that they are a part of the development process which af-fects their future.
d. Creates an environment which may later enhance the ac-ceptance of the service idea when it is formally launched.

Step Five: Concept Development and Refinement

The purpose of this step is to take all the inputs from the previous steps and develop alternative formulations of the basic concept. There will be a number of perspectives about the general features of a given concept or service idea. These alternative formulations of the concept should be tested with relevant groups to determine which formulations have the most merit.

For example, assume the development of patient service coordinators or a patient service center were being considered as a method of handling fear and ignorance of medicine and problems of processing patient admissions forms. It would be useful to test the alternative formulations by seeking the input of nurses and admissions personnel.

Step Six: Service Prototyping

As a result of the preceding steps, health service administrators should have a reasonably clear understanding of what service idea is most desirable. It then becomes important to translate the conceptual ideas into real service plans with detailed requirements—a prototype.

There may be a number of prototypes that can fit the general service idea. In some cases, the prototypes may not deliver all the characteristics a potential user would desire as part of a service offering, hence requiring a charge. For example, assume "home style" child delivery service (that is a birthing room versus separate labor and delivery rooms) is under consideration. This service should be tested before costly conversion to permanent facilities is done. Developing a prototype may also indicate what additions or alterations need to be made to make that service suitable.

In other cases, the prototypes might exceed the expectations created by the service idea. For example, it is possible to "over-engineer" a piece of equipment or a facility such that it handles much more than is required or suggested by the service idea. In these cases, a perfect matching of the prototype with the service concept is missing.

For these reasons, it might be useful, in some cases, to test the prototypes separately from the refined service concept to determine potential users' reactions to the prototype.

Step Seven: Match the Service Idea with the Prototype

Ideally it would be nice if the best prototype matched the best service idea. Unfortunately, frequently there is a mismatch (i.e., one cannot deliver all the expected benefits or one undersells the actual perceived value of a service). The purpose of this step is to test both the service ideas and the actual service plans (prototypes) to determine which alternatives offer the best match.

This step helps remove the flaws in a program and helps to refine the whole service plan. It also helps to establish boundaries as to the appropriate and believable public relations stances the health service may want to test. This step serves as a useful input for developing communications pieces which will position the service in the minds of the potential users.

Step Eight: Develop and Refine a Program for Communicating the Service

The testing completed in the earlier steps will identify the important service benefits and what features are easily understood. The benefits of the service need to be clearly recognizable because the perceivable benefits will serve as the mainstay of any communications program. The positioning of these benefits in the minds of the potential user of the health service is crucial.

This step may appear too simple to be considered as a separate step. However, the potential for miscommunication or poor communication is great and the anticipation of these problems is very important. Consider the difficulty of communicating the merits of a new preventive (not early diagnosis) health service. While few disagree about the worthwhile nature of the concept, few individuals are committed enough to alter their life styles to obtain the advantages. However, some specific service benefits have a greater appeal to certain groups of people than to others. Consequently, the communication of these benefits which have great appeal will be relatively easy. However, those benefits with more complex appeals will need more creative thought given to the communications. These communications need to be developed and tested to determine the best one to use for the desired target group.

Once the desired communication positions are established, a communications theme and a number of alternative communications pieces need to be developed for each communications medium that will be used. The best execution for each medium should be selected keeping in mind that the consistency and continuity between each medium is desirable. This means advertising, public relations releases, brochures, pamphlets, flyers and all other related communications should present a unified theme to the specific target group.

Step Nine: Testing the Complete Service Program

Before a new service is put into full scale operation it is usually desirable to test market, i.e., execute a demonstration project. Demonstration projects are commonplace in the health care sector.

A good example of testing an innovative service can be found in an article titled "Mobile Center Links Providers with Isolated Senior Citizens."[9] It describes how understanding the needs of the target group (senior citizens) led to the development of a new service and how the service was tested to determine its acceptance by the target group.

In this testing stage, a complete plan involving marketing and non-marketing functions is developed to ensure that proper staffing, facility availability, supplies and other needs are available when needed. A demonstration project should reveal the strength and weakness of the new service program. Program goals should be identified and measureable if possible. Provisions should be made for monitoring the successes and failures of the program. Adjustments should be made where needed and suggestions should be made to improve the program when it is put into full scale operation.

Step Ten: Certificate of Need Application

One element in the implementation of new services for the health care industry which adds a level of complexity not always found outside the health industry is the need for local, state and federal approval. This approval mechanism requires a "Certificate of Need." New health service programs must have an application showing there is a demonstrable need for the program in order to obtain local, state, and federal approval and meet the requirements of P.L. 93-641.

This document has been the target of much consternation for many energetic groups who are trying to improve the delivery of health services. Rejection by decision-making groups like the local Health Systems Agencies who "just don't seem to share the same points of view" produces much frustration. The process suggested here may help provide support information, validate the viewpoints and demonstrate the extent of patient needs to be satisfied by a new service presented in a certificate of need.

Step Eleven: Full Scale Introduction of New Service

The evaluation of the demonstration project should lead to refinements in the overall introductory program for the new service idea. Usually, the refinements will be minor adjustments to the demonstration project plan if the original plan was well conceived and executed.

The introductory plan should keep in mind that the new service may have a limited life cycle. Consequently, it is important to develop a life cycle maintenance program which involves: monitoring the performance of the new service over time, making changes to maintain effectiveness of the service, and phasing out the program when its usefulness is past. This monitoring system should be an integral part of a continual adjustment program to prolong the useful life of the new service.

IMPLICATIONS

The effectiveness of the eleven step process just described will vary depending on the environment of the organization into which it is introduced. All of the steps of the process will help to enhance the successful development of health services thus increasing acceptability by potential users. It should be noted that the process is useful not only to design services for patients or consumers of the system but also for designing services for internal staff.

Another benefit of the process described is that it is facilitated by and contributes to long-range planning by pinpointing changes and trends in the target market. The process establishes a priority for projects and provides for periodic reassessment of services. One benefit that may be more apparent is the noticeable sequence of steps that leads to a specific recommendation for a service. This process is aimed at gaining a Certificate of Need and producing well received services.

SUMMARY

This article presents an ideal sequence of steps to take in creating and developing new services. Health delivery systems face sizeable economic and social costs. The introduction of new services helps the delivery system keep in touch with changing consumer needs but represents a high risk situation (especially in light of the Certificate of Need requirement). This article does not attempt to present detailed substeps that vary from system to system and project to project. Rather it attempts to present a paradigm which can be modified to fit the needs of each specific system. It may be viewed as a means to reduce risk by providing a method of creating services the consumer will accept and use.

NOTES

1. "Current Business Statistics," *Survey of Current Business,* December 1976, pp. 6–14.

2. *Management of New Products,* 4th ed. (New York: Booz, Allen & Hamilton, Inc., 1965) p. 11.

3. O'Meara, J. T., Jr., "Selecting Profitable Products," *Harvard Business Review,* January-February 1961, p. 83.

4. Schorr, B., "Many New Products Fizzle, Despite Careful Planning, Publicity," *Wall Street Journal,* April 5, 1961.

5. Robert Byrne, "Users Point the Way to Best Hospital Design," *Modern Hospital,* vol. 113, no. 5 (November 1969) pp. 108–111.

6. Haynes, Warren, and Massie, Joseph L., *Management: Analysis Concepts and Cases,* 2nd ed. (Englewood Cliffs, N. J.: Prentice Hall, Inc., 1969) p. 236.

7. Osborn, Alex F. *Applied Imagination,* 3rd ed. (New York: Charles Scribner's Sons, 1963) p. 156.

8. For an example of this service see Gavin, Marshall P. "Consumer Services: Inhospital Recchant," *Hospitals, J. A. H. A.,* vol. 49 (July 16, 1975) pp. 65–67.

9. Stuart, Marian R. and K. J. MacKay, "Mobile Center Links Providers with Isolated Senior Citizens," *Hospitals J. A. H. A.,* vol. 52, (January 1, 1978) pp. 101–105.

23. The Birth of a Service: Conceived by the Patient, Delivered by the Hospital

C. T. HARDY AND LAMAR EKBLADH, M.D.

Adapted by the authors from an article originally published in *Hospitals, Journal of the American Hospital Association* (Vol. 52, March 2, 1978). Copyright 1978, American Hospital Association.

The North Carolina Memorial Hospital is a state supported institution affiliated with the University of North Carolina Medical School. Over the past decade, the OB service at this hospital has handled approximately 1,000 deliveries per year. Drawing its patients from all over the state, as well as the university community in which it is located, this service has always dealt with a diversity of patients despite its low census.

Background

The O.B. Service at North Carolina Memorial could be categorized as "liberal" throughout its history. Fathers in the delivery room, rooming-in of infants, childbirth techniques such as Lamaze and Bradley have been practiced there for a number of years. This has been due to both the patient population demands and the interest of the staff. All Delivery Room personnel are familiar with these procedures and have been involved in their formulation.

The hospital administration is organized in such a way that team work between the physicians, nurses and administration is formally used in operating all patient care areas of the hospital. This Triad concept has allowed the administration not only to deal with its staff in a positive, involved way, but has broadened its channels of communications with the patients. It was through this formal Triad system of weekly meetings between an O.B. physician, the R.N. in charge of the Delivery suite and an assistant administrator in charge of that service that a new concept in providing hospital deliveries was developed.

Two reflections of patient demand became apparent to the Triad concerning the delivery service, and they appeared to be strong enough to require a significant response. In fact the medical staff was very concerned about patient welfare. The cause of these demands was a growing popularity and interest in "home-style" delivery.

The first type of patient demand was the most dangerous to that group. This was reflected in several admissions of women and children who had gone through a home delivery. The problems encountered by this group were serious and could have been avoided by a hospital delivery. The medical staff was appalled that despite these complications, the parents were almost 100% in favor of home deliveries postpartum. It was also of concern that those admissions only reflected a percentage of persons actually going through a home delivery, either without or with an undetected complication.

The second reflection of demand appeared through a significant number of patients who made requests, often actual demands, that would minimize the institutional and medical aspects of their care. Patients presented the obstetrical staff with lists of "dos and don'ts" ranging from which types of medications should be used during delivery to whether or not the mother and child should be separated immediately after delivery. These demands were generated from "home-style" delivery philosophy and training; and they created various problems for the staff.

Professional training and experience, hospital routine, available facilities, laws concerning the care of newborns and other factors all presented difficulties in responding to this patient demand. The Delivery Room found itself dealing with hostile patients, families, instructors and friends who felt they were inflexible. This hostility was hard for the staff to deal with and created several bad situations.

In order to meet and resolve this problem, a committee was formed to deal with the potential conflicts of the situation. This committee consisted of representatives from the departments of obstetrics/gynecology, family medicine, and pediatrics; the labor and delivery suite; the maternity floor staff, the hospital administration; and the house staff. It also included, as consumer representatives, a husband and wife who were expecting a child and who desired delivery at home. The committee investigated the means through which the obstetrical service and the hospital could deal with the desires of the patients and, at the same time, maintain the benefits of the medical and institutional environment.

New Maternity Room Care

After discussing the various positions of the individuals on the committee, it was agreed that deliveries should take place in the hospital environment. The committee came up with the idea of a home-style delivery room—a facility within the hospital in which a woman could go through labor and delivery in surroundings that were more like a bedroom at home than a hospital delivery room. The key was that this room retained the benefits of hospital care.

The primary discussion on this room centered on whether it should be isolated from the labor and delivery suite or not. The fact that such isolation would defeat the hospital's purpose to respond to consumer demand without compromising the benefits of the hospital environment was debated. This discussion convinced the consumer representatives that the hospital and its staff were sincerely interested in meeting their needs and in responding to their ideas. Therefore, it was determined, and the consumer representatives concurred that one of the hospital's three labor rooms could be converted into the home-style delivery room. This arrangement would have several advantages in that:

1. The room could be provided with a less institutional appearance by applying some paint and wallpaper rather than by removing tile and surgical lights or making other major changes;
2. The room was large enough to accommodate a standard bed instead of a labor room bed and to house other furniture for the comfort of the patient and her visitors;
3. Medical gas outlets and other equipment and facilities that might be needed during a delivery would be available; and
4. If the demand on the labor and delivery suite required additional beds, this room easily could be reconverted to a two-bed labor room.

It was proposed that the small equipment, instruments, and trays that are used during delivery be stored in the vanity under the sink. However, the nursing staff and house staff members expressed concern regarding the instruments required, the location of equipment, and the techniques to be used in the home-style delivery room. The senior medical staff members, who provided care to most of the patients interested in this type of facility, believed that small equipment items could be concealed until they were needed, although they did not agree with the consumer representatives on the degree of concealment that would be appropriate. After much discussion, a compromise was reached. The large pieces of equipment are concealed behind the curtain, some small items are stored under the sink, and most of the items are stored on a cart that is moved into the room at the appropriate time. This solution allowed more equipment to be available for use in deliveries without detracting from the atmosphere of the room.

It was decided that a standard hospital bed would be used in this room. With the side rails removed, several additional pillows and an attractive bedspread, this bed resembled a large single, nonhospital bed. In selecting the bed, consideration was given to cleaning needs and the possible need for use of stirrups during delivery.

The remaining furnishings for the room included a large vinyl-covered rocking chair, a vanity sink, a pole lamp, and various wall hangings. All of the furnishings were selected for comfort, ease of cleaning, and practicality. A curtain was placed inside the entrance to the room, so that the door could be opened without disturbing the atmosphere in the room. This curtain also conceals an infant warmer and other larger pieces of equipment that might be needed during delivery.

Policies and procedures for the home-style delivery room were determined by the committee. It was felt that this facility would be used by low-risk patients who are not expected to require any unusual procedures or care during labor and delivery. A patient and her physician should make the decision to use this room during the patient's pregnancy, and that decision is noted on the patient's prenatal chart. Final confirmation is made at the time of the patient's admission, based on the risk assessment made during the admission physical examination. The new rules further required couples who are interested in using the home-style delivery room to attend some type of childbirth preparation class. The staff makes information on such classes available to them. If two patients arrive to use the home-style delivery room during the same period, it is assigned on a "first come, first serve" basis.

The number of visitors in the labor and delivery area created conflict between the consumer representatives and some of the hospital staff members. The physical facilities could not accommodate any major increase in the number of people in the labor and delivery area. This situation was the primary consideration in placing the limitation on the number of visitors. Infection control also was an important consideration. An alternative that is being pursued is the development of a new labor and delivery area that will be completed in three to four years and that will be designed to eliminate these limitations. However, it was decided the two persons of the patient's choice may remain in the room throughout labor and delivery. Patients who use the regular labor and delivery suite are still limited to one visitor.

A number of things were considered in the development of the policies. For example, sibling visitation in the labor and delivery area and on the rest of the maternity floor was strongly promoted by the consumer representatives. However, it was determined that the area's physical layout made sibling visitation difficult to monitor in order to ensure infection control. An alternative that is being pursued is the development of a family room, located near the maternity floor, where siblings can visit their mothers and their newborn brothers or sisters.

The number of medical procedures to which both the mothers and the newborns are subjected was considered too high by the consumer representatives. However, after discussion about what "routine" procedures are and why they are performed, very few of them were changed. The committee found that, for the home-style approach to be effective, the patients needed to have good communication with their physicians concerning the hospital and its policies prior to labor and delivery rather than many policy changes concerning medical care. Any individual concern could be dealt with in this way.

The patient charges for use of the home-style delivery room are the same as those for use of the rest of the labor and delivery suite. It is not anticipated that this type of delivery will require more staff time for patient care, use of more nonchargeable items, or more procedures. The initial cost of establishing the room was not significant and will be recouped through the anticipated increase in the volume of maternity patients.

The Success of the New Service

This new home-style delivery room has not only served to respond to a patient demand, it has also proven to be a stimulator to the number of deliveries. The increase in deliveries from 1976 to 1977 was 3.4% for a total in 1977 of 1,318 deliveries. Between December 1977 and December 1978, an increase of 10.8% is reflected in the '78 figure of 1,460 deliveries. The home-style delivery room got into full swing in June of 1978, and 75 deliveries were completed there before the end of December. This reflects 10% of half of the 1978 deliveries. In January of 1979, fifteen out of 143 deliveries were completed in the home-style delivery room. All 90 home-style deliveries have been accomplished without major complications.

As would be expected, some initial problems developed in opening this room. Guidelines were written in language that was too restrictive and created a situation in which the nurses felt uneasy about using the room for any purposes other than home-style deliveries. This situation caused unnecessary overcrowding in the other labor rooms. However, revision of the wording of the guidelines and personal communication quickly eased the problem. Consequently, the room now also is used for labor or monitoring without home-style deliveries, when this is necessary.

Although no formal announcement was made or publicity conducted about the home-style room, the medical staff members have received many requests for use of this room. The hospital apparently did respond to a real need of its patient population and benefited by increased deliveries. Because the committee was composed of representatives who believed in the extreme points of view of their groups, many of the issues and challenges involved in the project were faced and resolved before the home-style approach was used in a patient care situation.

The Triad format of the hospital administration was expanded to include consumers, and by dealing with the heated issues early, many points of conflict, misunderstanding and reservations were overcome before the room was actually functioning. The same effect the hospital had experienced in dealing with its staff took place with the consumers. Further, a good format for the one-to-one patient/physician relationship was established.

MARKETING RESEARCH AND MARKETING INFORMATION SYSTEMS

OVERVIEW

This section introduces the concept of marketing research and marketing information systems for the health care industry. Marketing research is a support function and can be done for each of the four areas: Consideration, Access (or Availability), Promotion, or Service Development. The purpose is to supply information for market planning purposes. Generally, this activity revolves around gathering information outside the organization. Many times the discovery that such information is needed is a reaction to a problem, and little planning and little or no budget allocation has been made. The result is that the research is conducted on a shoestring. Research for new medicine is planned and well-financed and provides significant findings. Research for health care marketing planning also should be planned and financed well if significant and reliable results are to be expected. The first article, "Marketing Health Care: Problems in Implementation," discusses the place of marketing in the health care field, introduces the problems of marketing research, and reviews the consequences of doing that research on a shoestring budget.

Gathering data on a continuing basis from inside the organization calls for the development of a marketing information system. The integration of all marketing functions was mentioned before and will be again in the last reading. Perhaps the most valuable tool to perform this integration function is the marketing information system. It can contain a variety of data ranging from a continuing patient attitude measure to a weekly review of the number of persons involved in delivering a particular service. The information gathered is dependent on the objectives and goals of the organization. The second article, "Marketing Your Hospital," briefly discusses marketing for hospitals, reviews three major segments (physicians, community, and government), and introduces the concept of marketing information systems.

The last two articles, "Discovering What the Health Consumer Really Wants" and "Marketing Assures a Satellite Facility a Safe Send-off," both include examples of health care marketing research. The first describes a specific type, "focus group research," and how it can be used to develop health services. The second discusses a market research study conducted for the Evanston (Ill.) Hospital. It shows how marketing research provides the input and feedback to direct efforts in planning for change.

24. Marketing Health Care: Problems in Implementation

ROBERTA N. CLARKE

Reprinted from *Health Care Management Review* Vol. 3, no. 1, Winter 1978, by permission of Aspen Systems Corporation, © 1978.

Most health professionals who have cast a sideways glance at marketing have recognized its value and, rather than asking "should we or shouldn't we?" now ask "how do we implement marketing in our organization?" Here's how to handle the implementation of a marketing program and a sampling of what to expect.

The advent of PSROs, Utilization Review Committees and the general decline in patient days had led to a problem of overbedding in hospitals and other institutional health care facilities. In addition, the availability of "easy" money in the 1960s allowed both the development of a large number of health facilities such as neighborhood health centers and the expansion of existing hospitals, which had not been forced in their early stages to consider whether sufficient demand existed to keep their organizations alive when soft money was no longer available.

MARKETING: ONE SOLUTION

The soft money is gone and some health care organizations are now faced with the problem of empty beds and vacant waiting rooms. One solution that has been suggested to alleviate this problem is marketing: marketing to attract patients, marketing to attract physicians, marketing of the more profitable health care services.

Discussions of marketing as an appropriate component of health care management have now reached the stage where health care professionals rarely ask: is or is it not appropriate? Most health professionals who have cast a sideways glance at marketing have recognized its value and, rather than asking "should we or shouldn't we?" with regard to the use of marketing, are now posing two different queries: (1) what exactly is marketing as applied to health care? and (2) how does one implement marketing in a health care organization?

Marketing Applied to Health Care

The first question has been addressed in a number of articles, in marketing textbooks and in conferences and symposia. Much of this explanatory literature addressing marketing in health care has been written by marketing academicians with limited exposure to the health care system rather than by practitioners. It therefore tends to assume a pedagogical tone with a traditional marketing emphasis on product, price, promotion and place, etc. The academic approach notwithstanding, this appears to be the most reasonable way to explain the concepts of marketing as they apply to health care.

Implementing Health Care Marketing

The second question—how does one implement health care marketing?—is the more difficult one to answer. The difficulty lies not so much in the answer itself as in the practical problem of implementation. The implementation of a marketing strategy for any health care organization is dependent, in each case, upon the specific situation (the particular organization, consumer population, competing providers, etc.). However, there are certain practical problems which are readily generalizable across most health care organizations when it comes to the inclusion and implementation of marketing in health care management.

PROBLEMS WITH MARKETING IN HEALTH CARE

Lack of Training and Background

There are few health care managers (excluding some in HMOs) with any training or background in marketing. The traditional professional degrees which were supposed to provide preparation for entry into health care management positions were the masters of public health (MPH), of hospital administration (MHA), of public administration (MPA) and the like, none of which include marketing in their curricula. Additionally, managerial positions in health care are often filled by physicians whose formal training not only lacks a marketing component, but often includes a chastisement of those availing themselves of the promotional benefits of marketing. (The value and the future of the AMA antisolicitation rule has been the subject of much controversy.) The results have been, at worst, a distrust of marketing and, due to a lack of understanding of just what marketing is, a failure to recognize the value of marketing to health care institutions. More frequently, health care managers with no marketing training have learned from brief explanations that marketing would be a useful function within their organizations, but they do not know how to incorporate marketing expertise into their organizational structure.

No Administrative Position for Marketing

In community hospitals and neighborhood clinics representing a major portion of the health care providers in this country, where top nonmedical management is the administrator—and middle management consists of the administrator's secretary—there is no administrative position into which a health care marketer fits. Even in major hospitals of substantial size, the various managerial positions have been allocated to individuals with traditional health care management skills; marketing has not been one of these skills. To force fit a marketer into an organizational structure not designed with a marketer in mind would be disruptive. (This is not to say that this is impossible, but rather likely to be avoided.)

Because health care managers rarely have a marketing background and cannot easily acquire marketing expertise within their organizations, the outcome is that they may not recognize a marketing problem when they are faced with one and that they may not recognize the value of the marketing function to health care management. If they do, they may have difficulty incorporating marketing into their organizations.

Solutions

There appear to be three solutions to this problem on an immediate basis. One is to make available to health care managers marketing courses, seminars or conferences geared to their organizations or to the health care system. There are few of these courses yet offered; most existing marketing courses do not make applications to the health care field. However, the number of health care marketing courses and seminars are on the increase.

Secondly, health care organizations may seek to hire experienced managers from outside the health care field for their managerial positions. These individuals, in addition to offering managerial experience, are also likely to have training, experience or both in the field of marketing. The quality of this second solution is highly dependent upon the skills and abilities of the individual manager. The drawback to this solution is that experienced managers from outside the health care field will need a substantial amount of time to acquaint themselves with the peculiarities of the health care field (third party payment, regulations and regulatory agencies, the division of medical tasks between various types of providers, etc.) before being able to effectively manage.

Thirdly, one may temporarily hire marketing expertise on a consulting basis. This solution is primarily effective in addressing a specific marketing problem or set of problems.

Outside Consultants Can Help

For example, a medical rehabilitation center with a spinal cord injury unit found a long-term trend of underutilization of this unit. Therefore, the rehabilitation center called in an outside consulting team to make recommendations to increase the unit's utilization. The consulting team ascertained: (1) the number and nature of competitive spinal cord injury units in the same geographical area, and the number of patients served by these units; (2) the nature of the spinal cord injury services offered by the center, and the satisfaction with these services on the part of former patients, referring physicians and third party payers with some influence on the patient's choice of service unit; (3) long-term trends in primary demand (total size) of the market; and (4) the referral mechanisms by which potential patients were or were not referred to the specific spinal cord injury unit.

The consulting team was able to discover declining primary demand, a large number of other spinal cord injury units which were also underutilized and a competitive service unit nearby with superior resources, equipment and facilities, a higher staff/patient ratio, and an excellent referral system. Therefore, the consulting team recommended an action which the center itself may not have seen as quickly, had the recommendation been generated internally: that the center close its spinal cord injury unit, since it would be unlikely to counteract its underutilization trend; and that the center focus its resources on other offered services which faced less competition and for which there was yet unmet demand.

The use of outside marketing consultation can be very helpful in many situations, but its drawbacks must be recognized. The hiring of marketing expertise on a consulting basis can be costly. The consulting project for the rehabilitation center just described cost in the range of $6,000 to $8,000. Also, this alternative does not make the marketing function a part of the internal management structure, as it should be, but allows it to remain external to the organization.

The ideal but long-term solution, of course, is to educate future health care managers in the field of marketing during their professional training.

Function of Marketing Misunderstood

It is not yet understood within most parts of the health care system that marketing is a major policy-making function and therefore belongs in a top management or equivalent position. As it is, in profit-motivated businesses, marketing should be on an equal footing with the financial, planning, budgeting, labor management and operations management functions. In most health care organizations (again, to the exclusion of HMOs' prepaid group practices), it is not.

Often, marketing is lumped together with the public relations function under the mistaken assumption that marketing is equivalent to public relations. The public relations office is never a top management office. Because of their lack of familiarity with it, health care providers tend to view marketing as a "neat idea" with interesting potential — but as peripheral to top management decisions.

Contrary to this belief, marketing involves decisions basic to the nature of the organization: what services to offer (product policy), whom to serve and how (market segmentation, product/market match), issues of pricing referral and access. It is marketing, for example, which may be the function best able to address an issue facing many hospitals today: whether to close down departments within the hospital due to decline in demand, to attempt to stimulate selective demand, or to negotiate with competing hospitals for certain departments in exchange for others ("We'll take all of maternity and give you pediatrics").

Failure to Position Marketing Properly

An illustration of the failure to position the marketing function properly within the organization is that of a large city hospital which made the mistake of assigning the organization's marketing to a mid-level supervisor already overloaded with administrative tasks. Not only was the supervisor unable to spend adequate time analyzing the hospital's major markets and competitive stance, but also the supervisor found that he was unable to obtain support for the few (quite reasonable) marketing actions he recommended. Because no one in top management had initiated the analysis from which the recommendation came and no top level manager was responsible for the marketing function, no one with the power to implement the recommended marketing actions would support them. The result was a frustrated supervisor who spent a good deal of his overallocated time on a nonproductive task and a hospital which missed out on two substantial market opportunities.

An Interim Solution

It will be difficult in the short run to incorporate marketing into top management. The best alternative at present to facilitate the proper use of marketing is to invite marketing expertise in whatever form possible into the policy-making office within the organization on a consistent basis. On the other hand, a great disservice will be done to furthering the acceptance of marketing if it is inappropriately used on a patchwork and inconsistent basis by managerial levels without the authority to implement marketing strategy.

Local Political Conflicts

Marketing-based strategy decisions are frequently at odds with local politics, community and individual desires. Speculation as to why this is so would probably focus on individual and community subgroup goals vs. the organizational goals of the health care institution.

Community Desires Dictate Product Management

A currently common conflict which is a classic marketing issue when translated into product management terms is the hospital which is torn between maintaining or closing its underutilized maternity ward. Almost every community thinks it should have a full service hospital; having a full complement of community services plays a significant part in community pride and image. It also plays a role in the spirited competition between some neighboring towns; no town wants to place its real estate agents in the position of having to say to a prospective buyer, "We have a good hospital here, but you'll have to go to the neighboring town to have your baby." The desires of the community would thus dictate keeping an underutilized maternity ward open.

A marketing approach, on the other hand, would point out that a poorly used maternity service results in a higher mortality rate (with highly negative marketing implications in terms of word-of-mouth and bad publicity, as well as low repeat purchase), a higher overhead cost per birth, poor space utilization (particularly if another service is cramped for space) and very possibly an angry local health planning agency.

This is not to say that a decision based on a marketing analysis would necessarily advise closing the ward. There are marketing-based product managers, for instance, who have elected to maintain a losing product, because it is one of the many products under a family name. In these situations, the product managers have concluded that it is more important to maintain a full complement of family-branded products than it is to rid themselves of one losing product—and be incompletely represented in the market (i.e., Kraft Salad Dressings with no Kraft Blue Cheese Dressing). The hospital with an undertilized maternity ward represents a strangely analogous situation.

Nonetheless, in the case of the hospital, a cost/benefit analysis performed on the advantages of keeping vs. closing the maternity ward would more than likely result in a consideration of closing the ward. The marketing implications in terms of lost business to the other services of the hospital as a result of the closing of the maternity ward, if judged to be insignificant, would suggest that the hospital might find it advantageous to put the maternity ward space to other use—and would also place a marketing-based decision at loggerheads with the community board of directors and local politics.

Interference with Marketing Strategy

A second example of conflict between a marketing vs. a community subgroup orientation, which interferes with the implementation of marketing strategy in a health care setting, is the introduction by a hospital of a primary care unit into the community. From a marketing viewpoint, it may be clear that the community is underserved, that there is not a sufficient number of family or general practitioners in the area and that many people, lacking other access to the health care system, resort to inappropriate usage of the hospital emergency room as a source of noncrisis medical care. To return its emergency room to its proper purpose—the provision of emergency care—and to provide better nonemergency medical care for people with no other access to care, the hospital, making a rational marketing strategy decision, proposed to introduce a primary care unit.

The conflict within the community, as has been seen to happen in similar circumstances in the past, arises from local physicians who fear loss of their patients to the primary care unit. They perceive the primary care unit as representing a major competitive threat to their individual practices, even though the supply for primary care services is known to be far less than the demand. The conflict is made more complex by the possible presence of some of these physicians of the hospital's board of directors and by the fact that the physicians are likely to have staff privileges at the hospital, thereby representing a major source of patients for the hospital. Needless to say, in a situation such as this, significant problems arise in attempting to implement the desired marketing strategy.

Compromise is the Only Solution

No easy answer or trite response can deal satisfactorily with conflict of this nature. Given other steadily growing pressures upon health care organizations which threaten the organizations' very existences, it will be necessary under conditions of conflict for a compromise to be made between marketing and community politics, with survival of the organization being the ultimate goal. While not a totally satisfactory solution to either party in the conflict, the necessity to meet ever larger challenges to its survival will require a health care organization to increasingly call for compromises on all sides from all interested parties.

Market Research Necessary but Costly

Marketing costs money. The marketing concept, a basic tenet of marketing philosophy, proposes the consumer population or the market as the basis of the development of all marketing strategy. Therefore, if better knowledge of the consumer is needed in order to determine product policy (programs to be offered), access problems, price sensitivities, unmet consumer needs, etc., then market surveys or consumer behavior/market research would be recommended. And good market research is costly.

Alternatives

The tendency of many health care organizations, when they learn of the expense involved in market research, is either: (1) to stop right there—to continue managing as they have always managed without the advantage of the insights provided by marketing, rather than incurring the expense of market research; or (2) to try to perform the necessary market research cheaply, through the use of volunteers, teenagers or work-study students and by decreasing population sample size, quality of survey, instrument design, etc. The problems inherent in this approach are manifold: there is enormous opportunity for bias to invade the development of a market research instrument; individuals without the expertise to recognize their own biases might elicit the results they want through exclusion of certain areas of questioning or by asking questions in biased ways.

Volunteers, lowly paid teenagers or students are generally poorly if at all trained; again, the opportunity for bias to enter the research exists and, at the very least, the collection of raw data is likely to be inconsistent and questionable. Lack of sufficient commitment on the part of volunteers *(et al.,)* whose responsibility it is to knock on doors or conduct telephone interviews results in their not putting in a sufficient number of hours to allow the research to be performed in a reasonable time period. At worst, a not-uncommon result is that research projects remain unfinished.

An Unsatisfactory Research Attempt

One example of this approach, of attempting to produce good extensive market research cheaply with typically unsatisfactory results, is a community hospital which intended to do a survey of its service area. In the hopes of saving money, the hospital enlisted the aid of an undergraduate work-study student with little training in the market research area to direct community volunteers in the performance of the survey. Fewer volunteers than had originally voiced interest actually became involved in the survey, which thus lost momentum not only because of an inadequate number of volunteer surveyors to cover the neighborhood but also because the work-study student spent little time on the project, recognizing that his commitment was over at the end of the semester, regardless of the state of the completion of the project.

An effort to complete the survey the following year, using teenagers sponsored by a federally-funded anti-poverty program as surveyors, also produced dismal results due to lack of commitment, training and ability of the teenagers. The newest plan of the hospital is to send a survey force of nuns into the neighborhood to administer the research questionnaire on a door-to-door basis. Such a survey force will eliminate some of the problems (commitment, interest) of the earlier volunteer groups, but will necessarily introduce bias into areas of the questionnaire dealing with alcoholism, venereal disease, abortion and birth control, at the very least.

The survey which this hospital wanted done could have been performed well and quickly by a consulting or market research firm experienced in this type of research. The cost for a survey of this nature varies according to the size and nature of the area to be surveyed as well as the firm involved. A reasonable estimate for this research effort is $15,000 to $25,000.

Negative Consequences of Unsatisfactory Research

Unfinished or questionable research results have negative consequences of their own. Having once performed poor market research, it might be more difficult to persuade those with funding power in the hospital to support a second (more expensive) better designed market research project; the consumer population might also be less willing to open their doors a second time as most market research represents an invasion of privacy.

Furthermore, it is reasonable to ask whether it is better to have no market research rather than to refer to dubious research results. Market research results often take the form of statistics which tend to have an implied legitimacy regardless of the nature of their birth. Most people, professionals included, view statistics as representing truth, soon forgetting that they questioned the method by which the statistics were produced. To have health care managers making major policy decisions based on misleading market research would seem to be less wise than to have them manage according to information gathered through their own informal management information systems.

No Reimbursement for Marketing Costs

Market research—as well as other marketing costs—are not reimbursed by third party payers. As the major financing mechanisms (Blue Cross, Medicaid, Medicare) introduce progressively more stringent reimbursement policies, it will become increasingly difficult for health care organizations to cover existing overhead, without even giving consideration to new and unprecedented marketing costs. It has become obvious to the most casual observer of the health care system that the financial squeeze upon all health care organizations is both great and growing; there is little "hidden" money available in most health providers' budgets to apply to experimentation in marketing. Until the major financing mechanisms recognize the value of marketing through their reimbursement policies, health care organizations will be reluctant to expend funds on marketing-related costs.

25. Marketing Your Hospital

RICHARD D. O'HALLARON, JEFFRY STAPLES, &
PAUL CHIAMPA

Reprinted from *Hospital Progress*, December 1976, Copyright 1976 by the
Catholic Hospital Association

Over the past 10 years, dramatic changes in population, competition, and government regulations affecting the health community have created problems for many hospitals throughout the United States. Projections of a 20 percent drop in inpatient census following the full implementation of professional standards review organizations is enough to cause any board of directors to think twice about the hospital's future. It is the purpose of this article to recommend that nonprofit hospitals with adequate financial resources create the position of director of marketing in order to deal with the problems at hand, to develop new sources of business and revenue, and to manage better the long-term growth of nonprofit hospital systems.

In profit-oriented industry the marketing director's role has traditionally been to deal with problems similar to those now faced by hospitals, and there is no reason why marketing as a discipline cannot be applied to nonprofit institutions. To support the case for such a position in the typical nonprofit hospital, the article will explore the different areas in which the marketing director might operate in order to demonstrate the utility such a position could have. The analysis will cover health care marketing in general, with special emphasis on marketing organization, marketing information services, and marketing research for the private nonprofit hospital. Hospital marketing may seem a novel concept, but it is one that can work.

At the present time, nonprofit hospitals engage in a number of activities which can be classified as marketing. Certain hospital personnel are responsible for employee relations, public relations, and other communications efforts inside and outside the hospital; many hospital auxiliaries mount fund drives and run various community activities; and the administration, in general, is responsible for long-range planning. Many activities carried out by various hospital departments, such as x-ray, laboratory, nuclear medicine, and emergency service, constitute marketing behavior. There is no apparent direction or coordination among these groups in most situations, however, that could ultimately pay off in greater awareness and use of hospital facilities by people in the area served by the hospital.

While planning is one key to a hospital's steady growth, a concerted effort to market the hospital and its services should be employed in order to maintain the superior image of the institution, to keep the public and physicians aware of the services the hospital has to offer, to insure the hospital's financial health, and to acquire both large and small charitable donations and funding from the many available appropriate sources which include individuals, private industry, foundations, and government. The marketing director would try to maximize these funding flows and would serve key hospital administrators as they need marketing and public relations assistance dealing with all their publics—patients, doctors, employees, and members of the local community.

Appointing a marketing director, improving the hospital's marketing information system, and directing more marketing effort toward other publics should benefit the hospital in several ways:

1. By increasing the flow of funds and volunteer interest in the hospital.
2. By improving the hospital's ability to meet the needs and wants of its patients, the community, and hospital visitors.
3. By attracting more and better physicians and other professionals to affiliate with the hospital.
4. By assisting in the development of long-range strategies and objectives.
5. By helping to answer questions related to allocation of resources and product pricing policies in order to insure a reasonable rate of return on investments.
6. By developing and overseeing the hospital's overall communications effort.
7. By dealing in an organized manner with local, state, federal, and regional planning and regulatory agencies.

The marketing director for a private nonprofit hospital would focus attention on four broad marketing areas which represent the relevant publics of a hospital: patients, physicians, the community, and government.

Patient Marketing

The hospital's first step in patient marketing is to define the patient population, since the nature of this market will influence the hospital's choices of services to offer, the doctors it will seek, and its potential sources of financial support. "With the patient market defined, a hospital has four broad options from which to select its own marketing orientation; i.e., it can choose a community orientation, a special public orientation, a research orientation, or a mix of these options."[1] In the past, many hospitals have been oriented to the community surrounding their hospital. The marketing director should assume responsibility for collecting information on population shifts in the area and changes in hospital usage by this population, in order to determine how these changes will affect the hospital, and recommend appropriate reactions to any significant changes found.

The key phases of a patient's experience with any hospital are (1) knowledge of services offered; (2) confidence in services offered; (3) admission to either inpatient or outpatient services; (4) exit from inpatient or outpatient services, plus contact through follow-up billing and repeat services.

The marketing director could work with nursing and administration to determine the level of care and satisfaction that should be rendered to patients in all service areas. "Dissatisfied patients can lead to an exodus of physicians, diminished benefactor support, and government agency intervention."[2] Since hospitals usually do not compete in this area of service, it could constitute an excellent opportunity for a hospital to gain a competitive advantage or distinctive competence.

Physician Marketing

Because most hospitals rely heavily on the medical staff to bring patients to the hospital, physician marketing becomes a vital area of concern for all administrative personnel. "This reliance on physicians creates two related problems: (1) attracting doctors to the hospital staff, and (2) making sure the doctors actually use the hospital's facilities once they are on the staff."[3] It is common for a hospital to grant privileges to physicians who have similar rights in three or four other hospitals in the vicinity. The hospital then finds itself very much in competition with other hospitals for the favor of these physicians. Many hospitals today are attempting to solve this problem by developing an office building for physicians adjacent to the hospital. Providing special equipment, such as gamma cameras, cardiac diagnostic equipment, and CAT scanners, special radiology diagnostic services, nuclear medicine, ultrasound, radiation therapy, and special care facilities, is another means used to lure physicians to a particular institution. The marketing director could serve as consultant to both a medical director and an administrator in determining what new services should be offered both to attract doctors to the hospital and to increase the utilization of the hospital's personnel and facilities. Developing an environment in which "a doctor wants to practice" is a highly important goal which requires sensitivity and coordination to achieve.

Community Marketing

"The purpose of community marketing is to develop close relationships between the hospital and the main organizations in the community."[4] Employees, volunteers, physicians, and patients all have community ties which should be exploited in the most effective manner possible. The marketing director should also maintain close contact with representatives of local media to promote news coverage of the hospital's programs and activities. An individual in this position should be prepared to disseminate pertinent news and information about the hospital via annual reports, publications, and personal appearances, and in addition this person must organize the hospital's means for gathering information on community health needs and perceptions and for providing health education programs to the community. A strong marketing information system is seldom seen but sorely needed in all health/hospital situations today. The marketing director's function is not only to increase the hospital's frequency of contacts with outsiders but also to ensure that the hospital projects a consistently professional image to the people it wishes to attract.

Governmental Agency Marketing

The full impact on the health care system of PL 93-641, the National Health Planning and Development Act, will probably encourage hospitals to set a high priority on the concept of a recognized marketing director for three reasons:

1. PL 93-641 has teeth—congressional guidelines must be followed—and to a significant degree requires the "quasi" use of the rules of evidence in its hearings and review of various projects and programs. In other words, the decisions of the local health systems agency (HSA) boards and the state health coordinating council must be logical and based on the presentation of hard facts. An HSA that makes politically motivated decisions contrary to the facts presented to it will surely be challenged in the courts, and its decisions will not be upheld.

    In the future, hospitals must know where they are, where they are going, and where their competition is if they are to obtain approval for their requests from local and state comprehensive health planning agencies and to succeed in developing new programs. A good marketing information system will help them accomplish these goals.

2. In the future, PL 93-641 will play a very important role in the evaluation of existing services in all hospitals throughout the country. A smart hospital executive, therefore, will want someone on the staff who is both interested in and able to monitor clinical service usage within the institution and community.

3. The health planning and development law has two major parts. One involves planning, coordination, and review of existing programs, and the second requires aggressive efforts to develop and organize new systems for the delivery of health care in each region. The marketing director could assist department heads, physicians, and administration to clearly conceptualize innovative ideas which are in their minds and hearts and also help them gain acceptance for these innovations. The hospital has the talent necessary to develop new ideas and new systems, but the handling of day-to-day problems keeps administrators from sitting down and completely thinking through many of their ideas for improving the various types of care the hospital delivers. The marketing director could pull together these thoughts, translate them into coordinated programs throughout the community, and fulfill a very important role in regard to PL 93-641. . . .

Marketing Information Systems

Various managers within a hospital may have very specific marketing information requirements. In order to design an internal record system, the marketing director would query a cross section of manager-users about their informational needs. Of ultimate importance to an information system are questions related to the types of decisions these managers make and the information they think they need to make these decisions. When opinions have been gathered, the director can proceed to design an efficient internal record system that reflects (1) what managers think they need, (2) what managers really do need, and (3) what is economically feasible.
(3) what is economically feasible.

Such information might include a list of potential donors, data on the activities of rival hospitals, and a forecast of future economic conditions affecting the hospital. Hospital personnel should be given incentives to pay more attention to gathering and passing along information to the marketing director.

The research assistant is essential to the marketing director in carrying out this information service and in conducting the necessary marketing research studies. The research assistant should determine market characteristics and market potential, analyze market share and sales, study competitive products and new product acceptability and potential, engage in shortrange forecasting, study hospital trends, and keep aware of governmental and health planning activities at multiple levels.

In summary, hospital administrators need timely, accurate, and easily retrievable marketing information if they are to make intelligent marketing decisions, and this information can be supplied by an active marketing department.

Qualifications for Position

The type of person needed to fill the role of marketing director should be one who is a self-starter, has leadership ability, relates well with people, has a basic understanding of marketing and management, and has a facility with statistics. This individual must have some degree of sales orientation and a willingness to learn and work. It should not be difficult to find well-qualified people who could evolve the marketing programs described in this article.

Such an individual is typical of many of the young people graduating from colleges and universities every year. An individual with a bachelor's degree in marketing or a master's degree in related subjects with an ability to write would be an excellent candidate. The level of students and the range of subjects they cover in the normal course of a university education in some of this country's higher quality schools are impressive. It takes a highly motivated person to handle all these subjects, and many such graduates would be willing to enter the hospital system at reasonable salaries. A person qualified as marketing director would be comparable in age, responsibility, training, and knowledge to many key managers presently in hospitals.

Conclusions

The typical nonprofit hospital faces many of the same problems which challenge larger, profit-oriented businesses and organizations in terms of a changing consumer, a more competitive environment, and increased governmental regulation. Unlike these organizations, however, most hospitals do not have an effective mechanism for dealing with such problems. Traditionally, demand for hospital facilities far exceeded the supply so that it was not important to think of such matters. As this supply-demand relationship begins to shift, marketing factors become all the more important and should be handled.

Marketing as a concept is novel to hospital administrators, although marketing behavior is not. Marketing activities carried on by a marketing director, rather than being antithetical to the goals of a nonprofit hospital, should be seen as a tool by which the hospital's administration can more effectively reach its goals of providing more and better care to the patient at a price he can afford.

NOTES

1. Philip Kotler, *Marketing for Nonprofit Organizations,* Prentice-Hall, Inc., Englewood Cliffs, NJ, p. 308.

2. Ibid., p. 310.

3. Ibid., p. 312.

4. Ibid., p. 314.

26. Discovering what the Health Consumer Really Wants

WILLIAM A. FLEXNER, CURTIS P. MCLAUGHLIN, AND JAMES E. LITTLEFIELD

Reprinted from *Health Care Management Review*, Vol. 2, no. 4, Fall 1977, by permission of Aspen Systems Corporation, © 1977.

A major theme to emerge from the 1976 presidential campaign was "Let's make government more responsive to the people." In health this is a challenging and often frustrating task. Consumer representation and consumer advocacy have been used, but they still leave a nagging doubt as to what is really wanted by a cross section of consumers or by special groups of consumers. One approach is to use the tools of marketing research to look at the choices made by health care consumers. The example cited here is a study of how potential and actual consumers, as well as the providers, view the choice process for a specific service—abortion. It illustrates a specific approach to information gathering and the differences that can exist among these groups when they are studied in detail.

A MARKETER'S CONCEPT OF RESPONSIVENESS

A basic concept which governs a marketing point-of-view of responsiveness is exchange. "It calls for the offering of value to someone in exchange for value. Through exchanges, various social units—individuals, small groups, organizations, whole nations—attain the inputs they need. By giving up something, they acquire something else in return. This something else is normally valued more than that which is given up, which explains the motivation for the exchange."[1] This exchange concept does not require that a classical marketplace exist. Even "free" health care has a cost to its recipients in time spent, travel, risk, perceived loss of dignity, dependency, etc. The staff may receive the gratitude and improved functioning of the patients as a benefit in addition to their salaries and titles. When services are considered in reciprocal benefit terms, the need for the provider to under-

NOTE: The work from which this article was written was partially supported by the Jessie Smith Noyes Foundation through a grant to the Carolina Population Center, University of North Carolina at Chapel Hill.

stand the consumer becomes as important as the need for the consumer to understand what the provider has to offer.

Kotler concludes that:

> Marketing relies on designing the organization's offering in terms of the target market's needs and desires rather than in terms of the seller's personal tastes ... Local governments that design playgrounds or toll roads without studying the public's attitudes often find the subsequent level of public usage disappointing. Effective marketing is user-oriented, not seller-oriented ... Too often the public equates marketing with only one of its tools such as advertising. But marketing is oriented toward producing results, and this requires a broad conception of all the factors influencing buying behavior. A church, for example, may do no advertising and yet attract a large following because of other elements appealing to the public's needs.[2]

The example of health care marketing most cited in the literature is the enrollment process for group health plans or HMOs.[3] But it would be tragic if this problem and its implication of selling the consumer on something that may or may not be feasible and may or may not be desired, were to become the dominant view of marketing in health.

CONSUMER CHOICE AND CONSUMER BENEFITS IN HEALTH CARE

Consumer need (as defined both by health care providers and consumers) is traditionally viewed in terms of health or medical care requirements.[4,5,6] Health providers develop "products" that they believe respond to these requirements. These products are often viewed by providers as those elements of technology that the consumer comes to buy, including the technical skill of the provider, the technological capacity of the institution in which the provider functions, and specific tests, surgical procedures and regimens that are prescribed.

A full description of the "product" in health care is incomplete, however, unless it also includes the notion that the consumer expects to obtain certain benefits beyond the best technical quality from the product being purchased. Among these benefits are the consumer's desire or concern for physical comfort, social and psychological support, and considerably greater ease in purchasing the primary health product.

Identification of the attributes or benefits that are most important to the consumer in deciding to use health services and in choosing where to go to obtain them is becoming increasingly important as the consumer is provided greater opportunity to shop in the marketplace of health care. This opportunity has resulted from diversification in the modes of health service delivery in the United States. Today, the number of different ways that a consumer can obtain health services is extensive: in most large, urban areas, one can obtain health services from a solo practitioner, a single-specialty group practice, a fee-for-service multispecialty group practice, a prepaid multispecialty group practice, a health maintenance organization, a hospital emergency room, a hospital outpatient specialty clinic, a neighborhood health center, a public health clinic, and so forth. Furthermore, within many of these service delivery modes, the consumer often chooses among several alternative places or organizations. Effective health care planning requires information related to why and how such choices are made.

Alternative Techniques

To be responsive to consumer desires, health care managers need techniques to identify the benefits that guide the choices made by health consumers—techniques that can articulate directly with the planning process of the organization and are relatively simple to implement.

There are a number of approaches to studying the consumer's decision process. Basic to all of these is the survey, either quantitative or qualitative. Figure 1 charts these alternatives and gives a short description of each.

One Management Tool for Generating Consumer-Responsive Health Services

Focus group discussion is another qualitative technique used to learn what is on consumers' minds concerning a given subject.[7, 8] A representative group of consumers is brought together and the general subject is introduced. Then, using an informal process, these consumers are allowed and encouraged to express their surface and deep feelings about the subject of discussion in any way they desire. A group moderator attempts, in the most diplomatic manner possible, to keep the discussion focused on the topic previously introduced. However, the moderator does not enter into the discussion in any substantive manner. As many members of the group as wish to may enter into the discussion. It is an opportunity for the health care manager to learn

Figure 1 Alternative Approaches to Studying the Consumer Decision
Process

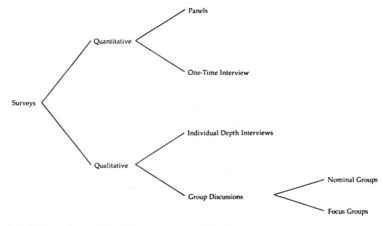

Quantitative *(telephone, mail or personal interview)*

— *Consumer panels* are groups of people studied longitudinally.
Replacements in the panels are made periodically to keep the
panels as "representative" as possible.
— *One-time questionnaires* are given to different groups of people
when specific questions need to be answered.

Qualitative

— *Individual depth interviews*, as the name implies, probe the decision processes of people one at a time.
— *Nominal group process* is a group discussion procedure used extensively in the health field.*

*Discussed in Delbecq, A.L., Van de Ven, A.H. and Gustafson, D.H. Group Techniques for Program Planning (Glenview, Ill.: Scott, Foresman and Co. 1975), and
McLaughlin, C.P., Sheldon, A., Hansen, R.C. and McIver, B.A. "Management Uses of the Delphi." Health Care Management Review 1:2 (Spring 1966) p. 51-62.

what is on the consumer's mind without influencing the respondent
with specific, structured questions, or closing the respondent out of
certain lines of thought.

Discussion is generated through the use of a focusing question. The
wording of the focusing question is critical to the success of the method.
Ideally, the question is prefaced with a few words about the context
within which the group participants should respond, followed by the
actual focusing question. Because the focusing question is so critical, it
is a good idea to pretest the question to be certain that it will generate
the appropriate discussion.

Results

The first product of a focus group discussion will generally be a series
of emotional and subjective statements that can be identified as elements of desires or requirements related to the problem under discussion. For example, in the area of what providers typically term accessibility or location convenience, such elements or phrases as "on a bus

route," "in a well-lighted area," "with controlled and ample parking facilities" and "with ramps instead of stairs" might come out in the discussion. The elements or phrases identified in the discussion form are, in effect, qualitative operational definitions of consumer benefits and can be used for further investigation into priority weightings, as will be discussed below.

At this point, the focus group discussion may arrive at a "surprising" conclusion as interpreted by the moderator or manager: in the example given above, the factor or benefit actually may be "safety" instead of "location convenience" per se. Thus, it is possible, even probable, that a new conception of how consumers perceive the process of obtaining health care will begin to emerge.

Because the number of respondents in a focus group discussion is small (eight to twelve), no numbers may be quoted, no generalizations may be made to the larger population from which the focus group sample was selected. In fact, if the population studied seems to have several ethnic groups or social strata, it may be necessary to conduct discussions within each of these groups or strata. This is qualitative research—research that attempts to identify the factors that can be given weights later.

Interpretation

After the focus group discussions have indicated the elements or phrases involved with consumer health benefits, it is then necessary to determine how important each of these is to the larger population from which the focus group discussion sample was chosen. This involves a two stage process beginning with a content analysis of the phrases to determine the range of benefits identified and concluding with the design and administration of a questionnaire or interview.

The object of this phrase of the research is to establish a weight as perceived by consumers for each benefit. In some cases these weights might be expressed as a priority ranking. Using the previous example, if the "benefits" discovered in the focus group discussion as related to "convenience of location," are actually divided into "distance" and "safety," then this second stage of the research can quantify the difference in importance between these two benefits.

Example

In a study just completed by one of the authors, the focus group procedures described above were used to identify the things that potential consumers, consumers and providers of abortion services felt were most important to a woman choosing where to go to get an abortion.[9] The following focusing question was used for the consumer group discussions (i.e., for women who had come to a facility for an abortion):

> This clinic is attempting to make its service as consumer-oriented as possible. One way of doing this is to get information directly from the women coming to this clinic. I would like to ask you a question to help us get some of this information. In answering, please don't worry at all about suggesting things that you feel should exist here. As I said, we are interested in providing the best service from your point of view. After you decided to get an abortion, what things were most important to you in deciding where you would go to get the abortion service?

The output of the focus group discussions was a series of phrases that were reviewed and categorized using a two stage content analysis procedure. Table 1 illustrates the types of phrases that were obtained during the group discussion. From the content analysis, eleven factors of concern to the respondents were identified. Using two phrases to represent differing aspects of each factor, a questionnaire was designed to collect information from the three respondent groups—potential consumers, consumers and providers—about the relative influence of the eleven factors on the choice of abortion services. Table 2 identifies the eleven factors and the phrases that were associated with each factor.

The major findings of the study were:

- **All three respondent groups** recognized the singular importance of the technical-medical factor. Beyond this, however, there were some important differences.
- **Potential consumers** were primarily concerned with obtaining general information about the physicians, the procedures used and their after effects, the standards for the facilities and the qualifications of the staff, and what the abortion facility is like.
- **Consumers** were concerned primarily with receiving an appointment right away and with the cleanliness, respectability, legitimacy and medical competency of the abortion facility and staff.
- **Providers** recognized that consumers were concerned about many of these issues, yet they failed to recognize the importance to the consumer of the facility being clean, respectable and staffed by friendly people.

Table 1   Sample Phrases Obtained from Focus Group Discussions

---

—Safety—lack cf adequate facilities
—Health—sanitary conditions
—Good doctor to examine me
—Also, counseling services for some support
—Confidentiality
—Time—wouldn't want to hang around for a week or so
—Two types of counseling—the emotional side & what repeated abortions would do to a woman's body—some risk involved
—Financial understanding—abortion insurance—something to help finance an abortion
—Adequate facilities for resting & if anything (problem) should arise
—Clinic have good relationship with hospitals
—Doctor should be on hand—absolutely want doctor on the spot
—Method—best way to be done
—Explain what is going to happen to you—exact prior knowledge
—Written materials—what are the standards—who are the doctors—what are their qualifications
—Sympathetic care from the receptionist through the doctor and counselor
—Training of staff—screen to see how they feel about abortions
—Preliminary appointment
—The atmosphere of the place
—Facilities comparable to a hospital
—Clinic attached to hospital

Table 2 Factors and Phrases Used in Questionnaires

    I.   Technical-Medical (TMED)
          Method used—best way to be done
          Make sure it was done safely by a doctor

   II.   Psychological-Supportive (PSYC)
          People have to be friendly
          Sympathetic care from the receptionist through the doctor
             and the counselor

  III.   Comprehensiveness (COMP)
          Other services are offered at same time as abortion
          Contraception introduced

  IV.   Future Health (FUTH)
          Follow-up physical checkup
          That I would be able to have a baby later on

   V.   Convenience (CONV)
          Location—availability
          Appointment right away

  VI.   Financial (FINA)
          Opportunity to make installment payments
          Initial thing is cost

 VII.   Physical (PHYS)
          Place that was clean
          Attractive—well laid out

VIII.   Privacy (PRIV)
          Confidential aspects—would it be kept secret
          Privacy—wouldn't go any place too close to me

  IX.   Informational Supportive (INFO)
          Written materials—what are standards; who are
             doctors; what are their qualifications
          Printed information on procedures and after effects

   X.   Referral Source (REFR)
          Doctor's recommendation
          Friend's recommendation

  XI.   Reputational (REPU)
          Respectable place
          Heard it was good place to go

Figure 2 Relative Importance of Factors Influencing Choice of Abortion Service

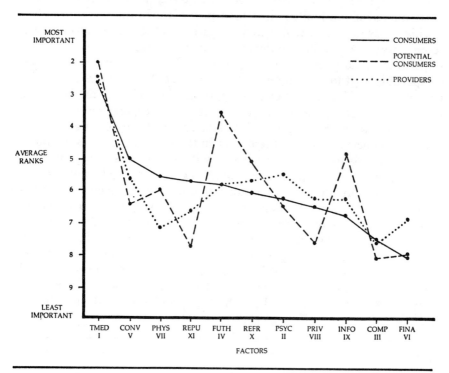

Figure 2 illustrates graphically some of the similarities and differences among the three groups.

Developing a Marketing Strategy

Using these findings a marketing strategy was developed. Elements of the strategy included (1) the design, production and distribution to referral agents and other interested parties, or groups, of an information brochure containing readable text and colored pictures to aid in the reduction of facility and procedure-related anxiety and stress, and (2) the establishment of an optional, immediate appointment procedure at the facility to provide information (including the brochure) about the process that the woman would go through on the day of her scheduled abortion. Furthermore, in addition to the positive effect that the brochure could have on the woman, use of the brochure by referral agents would stimulate them to recommend that their clients go to the particular abortion facility described in the brochure.

This study did not attempt to determine whether or not a consumer representative could have done as well at providing the data. But it is important to note that the study acquired, at little extra cost, the comparable attitudes of potential but not current consumers and of the provider staff. The utility of this approach depends on the degree to which it is used by health care managers to respond more fully to consumer desires. From a practical standpoint, by involving the consumers and providers from the outset in the research process, by holding separate focus group discussions with consumers and providers, and by avoiding preconceptions regarding the expected findings, the method can help indicate areas of agreement and disagreement between consumer and provider perceptions. Then, once these areas are determined, management can concentrate on resolution of the areas of disagreement. In that manner, with limited investment of resources, a health service can be designed that responds to the benefits identified by consumers as being most important. Such a health service should rapidly raise consumer satisfaction and could ultimately have an effect on future health behavior related both to prevention and compliance.

REFERENCES

1. Kotler, P. *Marketing For Non-Profit Organizations* (Englewood Cliffs, N.J.: Prentice-Hall 1975) p. 5.

2. *Ibid.*, 6–7.

3. Heyssel, R. M. and Seidel, H. M. "The Johns Hopkins Experience in Columbia, Maryland." *New England Journal of Medicine* 295 (Nov. 1975) p. 1225–1231.

4. Boulding, K. E. "The Concept of Need for Health Services." *Milbank Memorial Fund Quarterly* 44 (1966) p. 202–233.

5. Fuchs, V. "The Growing Demand for Health Care." *New England Journal of Medicine* 279 (July 25, 1968) p. 190–195.

6. Jeffers, J. R., Bognanno, M. F. and Bartlett, J. C. "On the Demand Versus Need for Medical Services and the Concept of 'Shortage.'" *American Journal of Public Health* 61 (1971) p. 46–63.

7. Goldman, A. E. "The Group Depth Interview." *Journal of Marketing* 26 (1962) p. 61–68.

8. Leonard, D. "Can Focus Group Interviews Survive?" *Marketing News* 9:6 (October 10, 1975).

9. Flexner, W. A. *Marketing Research and Health Care: Concepts and Techniques Applied to Abortion Service Design* (New York: Neale Watson Academic Publications, Inc.) Forthcoming.

27. Marketing Assures a Satellite Facility a Safe Send-Off

JOHN A. MCLAREN, M.D., AND
BARBARA S. TRAEGER

Reprinted, with permission, from *Hospitals, Journal of the American Hospital Association*, Vol. 51, June 1, 1977, pp. 67–69.

Marketing is commonly used in business and industry, but it is almost unknown in the hospital field. Until recently, only the most casual kind of marketing was being done by hospitals. Most hospitals have communications, or public relations, programs that reach their employees and service community, and most also directly solicit feedback from their patients. But only within the past two years have hospitals begun to embrace marketing formally.

Some hospitals are moving toward marketing because of lagging patient admissions. Others are turning to marketing in an attempt to strengthen referral patterns, and still others are considering it because they are planning to expand their physical plant. Whatever the reason, many hospitals are now becoming interested in marketing as a tool to maximize utilization of a variety of services, to identify needed programs or no longer needed ones, and to measure the effectiveness of their communications efforts.

Evanston (IL) Hospital has appointed a vice-president for marketing. With the creation of this position, a natural corporate sub-group has emerged, including marketing, development, and public relations. At the time of the appointment, the hospital was completing construction of a satellite facility, Glenbrook Hospital, located in Glenview, IL. The timing of the appointment underscores the commitment the hospital has made to expanding into a multihospital system and to acquiring 5,000 more patients per year when both hospitals are optimally utilized.

By placing its marketer at the vice-presidential level rather than at the managerial level, the hospital has ensured his participation at the meetings of the hospital's board of directors. This also ensures that he will be fully aware of the hospital's mission and of its plans for the future.

Planning Glenbrook

Both the Evanston Hospital and the Evangelical Covenant Church of America were interested in developing a hospital in the Glenview/ Northbrook area. In the late 1960's, the church's Board of Benevolence considered building a hospital on 22 acres of property in Northbrook. A comprehensive plan was prepared that proposed a phased development culminating in the establishment of an acute care general hospital. Some of the factors favoring the development of the hospital were also highlighted in the plan: The state plan of the Illinois Department of Public Health had identified District A6 (Northbrook) as one of two areas in the state in which a hospital was needed; Northbrook was in the center of an area of 70 square miles in which no hospital was located; and the surrounding township of Northfield was one of the fastest growing suburban areas in the Chicago vicinity.

In 1971, meetings were held between the Board of Benevolence and Evanston Hospital. As a result of these meetings, Evanston Hospital accepted the responsibility for the new hospital and agreed to keep in close contact with the Board of Benevolence to ensure that the original commitments to the community would be fulfilled.

The hospital then began to put together a plan of development. Demographic studies were compiled from data generated from two major sources—the Metropolitan Planning Council of Greater Chicago and the Northeastern Illinois Planning Commission. Studies of the four villages in Northfield Township were made according to population, size, density, biological characteristics, social characteristics, income, occupational status, marital status, and housing and educational levels. On the basis of these data, plans were developed for a 150-bed general hospital on a 40-acre site, and provisions were made to allow the hospital to expand to a maximum of 450 beds if needed in the future.

After meetings with the hospital's professional staff and further study of the Northbrook service area, including consideration of the role of other health care providers in the area, the hospital made some specific decisions regarding the makeup of the Glenbrook facility. Neither a maternity unit nor a radiation therapy unit would be developed. Initially, children and psychiatric patients would be admitted to general medical-surgical units until such time as patient volume would warrant the creation of separate care areas. These decisions having been made, the hospital began construction in December 1975.

Reaching the Community

Coincident with the start of construction, a major effort was begun by the development officer to raise funds and by the public relations director to increase the community's awareness of the new hospital. The development officer made a careful analysis of the population in the communities to be served by the hospital and learned that the residents of these communities are for the most part young, professional families with upwardly mobile lifestyles. Also residing in the area are a small, older, and more stable population and a small, highly transient population. Finally, we found that 25 percent of the population leave the area annually.

We then proceeded to differentiate the particular groups, or "publics," we wanted to reach using several criteria: age, income, church affiliation, and profession. We also divided the service area geographically and established priorities to guide us in our fund-raising and communications planning. Our initial challenge was to build a constituency within the communities we wished to serve. We did this through mass mailings and through the development of an introductory brochure containing a coupon to be returned indicating an interest in the new hospital. The coupon permitted the community's residents to choose the manner in which they would like to follow up on that interest. They could volunteer to raise funds, volunteer to work in the temporary office, or continue on the mailing list.

From the responses we received, we developed a corps of volunteers to help in the office and began to establish lists of our various publics. Lists were also developed by using customary fund raising techniques, such as the Haines Directory and poll sheets. The design and distribution of all of our communications tools, including our biweekly newsletter, slide presentations, brochures, displays, and posters, were dictated by the type of audience, or public, we wanted to reach.

Presentations before service clubs, churches, school groups, homeowner's associations, rotaries, and other community organizations were made by representatives of the hospital's public relations and development staffs and by the vice-president for Glenbrook. Our emphasis was on the family since our audience was, for the most part, family-oriented. The volunteer fund-raising group we developed demonstrates this emphasis; we sought out husband-and-wife teams to head each community fund-raising committee. Teenagers helped develop our float entered in the annual Fourth of July parades in these communities, and grandparents were among those who volunteered in the office. These efforts to get everyone involved paid off in several ways: We had a dependable corps of office volunteers working for us; the fund raising volunteers raised a good sum of money; and, perhaps most importantly, the communities came to identify the new hospital as their own.

While our approaches thus far had been sound and our results positive, it was apparent that it was time to examine new approaches and to set new goals based on the progress made to date. More input was needed from the community. Many questions still needed to be answered. How did the community's residents perceive hospitals and health care in general? What factors determined when, where, and how they sought health care? What did they know about the Glenbrook Hospital, its services, and its relationship to Evanston Hospital? Would they use it?

To try to answer these questions and others, the hospital contracted with the marketing department of Northwestern University in Evanston to do a market research study. Phase one of the market study identified four focus groups, with 10 to 12 people in each group. One-half of the participants were required to have been a hospital patient in the last five years. The other half could not have been a hospital patient in the last 10 years. The groups were almost equally divided by sex, and one-quarter of the participants were Jewish.

The results of phase one of the study have allowed the hospital to further clarify its role, or marketing "position," in the community. Certain aspects of that position are already established: Glenbrook is to be a teaching hospital; it is part of the McGaw Medical Center of Northwestern University; and it is owned and operated by Evanston Hospital.

To some extent, clarifying our position has meant clarifying our language. For example, many members of the focus groups did not understand "affiliated with Evanston Hospital," but were quite clear about "owned and operated by." "Not-for-profit" is another term that is not well understood. People believe that the hospital makes money and someone benefits from it. We need to be careful when we use this term and, whenever possible, we should try to make the community aware of its meaning.

The importance of the emergency department was also stressed by all of the focus group participants. An emergency visit is unscheduled and usually the patient has little control over his destiny. He needs to be assured that his care will be timely and of high quality. A highly active emergency department also provides the hospital with a means by which to help patients become established with a physician.

Phase two of the market research study will be a 24-page questionnaire designed to elaborate upon the information gathered from the focus groups. It will be sent to 1,000 families in the service area. Once the original data base is established, several methods will be used to keep it current. The most common method employed is that of direct customer solicitation by questionnaire. Sixty-five percent of all corporations engaged in marketing use this technique. It is well-tested and reliable.

Random telephone surveys also will be done monthly. Questions will test the community's awareness of the hospital, determine the potential and actual use of its services, and explore how patients go about seeking their physician or hospital. Today, more patients appear to be selecting their hospital first and their physician second, although twenty years ago the reverse was probably true. If this change is indeed taking place, it has important implications for hospital marketing.

Finally, the admissions information gathered by all hospitals gives valuable data on how well one is meeting the needs of various publics. The admissions process alone can produce patient profiles according to sex, age, religion, geographic location, admitting physician, and length of stay. At Evanston Hospital, this information is computer-generated on a regular basis and is enormously helpful to us in monitoring the character of our services.

The public relations plan will take direction from the research we now are doing. For example, brochures about the emergency department and how to best use it are now a high priority. We also need to consistently reiterate the relationships among the facilities within the Evanston Hospital system, including the place of the Glenbrook Hospital within that system, and tell members of the community how they can utilize these facilities to maximum advantage.

Although traditional development and public relations techniques proved effective at the time we used them, it is the input and feedback of marketing that is providing the criteria we need now, and it will continue to lend direction to our future efforts.

SECTION VI

HEALTH CARE MARKETING MANAGEMENT: ITS AUDIT, PLAN, AND STRATEGY DEVELOPMENT

OVERVIEW

This final section contains the essence of each of the previous sections and focuses on the integrative aspect of health care marketing. The previous articles discussed the health care marketing concept; consumer orientation; health care marketing C.A.P.S. (also referred to as the marketing mix variables)—Considerations (such as cost), Access, Promotion, and Service Development; and marketing research. Now it is time to tie them together with the development of a health care marketing plan.

Health planning traditionally has been an "inside out" process: an inventory is taken of what is available in the health planning area, this is matched with government guidelines, and steps are taken to adjust the situation and then inform the public. A health care marketing plan begins with the consumer or public and works back to the system.

The point needs to be made that the marketing audit and the marketing plan are events that need to be done on a periodic basis. It is an unfortunate fact that human beings rarely become involved in the expenditure of a lot of activity unless forced to. Health care is an excellent example of this problem. The major drawback in the development of preventive health behavior is the lack of a crisis to force behavior. Planning is not second nature. However, the crisis of inflation, the pressure of cost containment, and government regulations all increase the pressure for planning.

The logic of planning is obvious. Planning breeds efficiency in the use of resources. However, to plan properly takes time and resources. If the marketing audit and plan is done in a time of crisis, then resources necessary to do a good job usually are scarce. The crisis usually is a drastic drop in patient census or in the business sector—a drop in sales. In that event, funds are not available to do a thorough job and a patchwork audit and plan is the outcome. The marketing audit should be conducted and the marketing plan revised periodically. Any health care organization should plan or commit to plan periodically.

The first article, "Marketing Management: Health Care in General, Preventive Care in Particular," summarizes elements important to marketing planning, discusses market segmentation, and dwells on consumer analysis. The integration of the health care marketing mix variables (C.A.P.S.) is discussed in a preventive health care context. With the advent of HMOs and the pressure on cost containment, there is and will continue to be a move from horizontal (hospital-based) care to vertical (or ambulatory) care, thus increasing the importance of this context. Before a health organization can jump into the marketing planning process, it must take stock of its resources; the nature of the environment, its missions, goals, and sets of objectives; how the system is organized to meet the objective; the strengths and weaknesses of the health care marketing Mix elements; and many other issues.

The second article, "The Marketing Audit: A Tool for Health Service Organizations," describes a procedure for organizing and gathering marketing information as a necessary step before a plan or a strategy can be developed. Of all the tools a marketing approach can offer, a marketing audit is the most important in terms of planning.

The third article is an original manuscript designed to bring together the concepts spread throughout the book. The article, "Marketing: A New Opportunity for Hospital Management," is set in the specific context of the hospital that supplies a clear (and at this point the most popular) focus for health care marketing. It describes the health care marketing C.A.P.S. and the importance of the marketing audit. It ends with a discussion of the marketing plan or program and shows how the pieces fit together.

The last two articles have been developed especially for this book and are full of examples of health care marketing planning and strategy development. The article "The Use of Marketing Strategies in

Meeting Changing Needs," identifies investor-owned hospitals as excellent examples of the development of marketing plans, strategies, and the success of these methods. It looks at three examples: the full service hospital, the specialty hospital, and the expanded hospital.

The last article, "The Emergence of a Marketing Management Approach in a Time of Crisis," reviews the long-term effects of a marketing approach for a large hospital. It describes an almost five-year scenario. This hospital was lucky—it decided to develop a marketing plan before it was too late to plan.

28. Marketing Management: Health Care In General, Preventive Care In Particular

M. VENKATESAN

The complete article appeared as "Preventive Health Care and Marketing: Positive Aspects" in *Marketing and Preventive Health Care*, P.D. Cooper et al., editors. Reprinted with permission of the American Marketing Association, Chicago, Illinois. Copyright 1978.

Direction of marketing activities *is* the management of marketing in any organization. This generally involves three tasks, viz., (1) planning (strategies), (2) directing, and (3) controlling (evaluation and control). Formulating marketing strategies involves identification of target markets (often called "segments") and the development of a marketing plan, which is the selection and combination of "marketing mix variables". Identification and selection of appropriate market targets and the choice of instruments to be coordinated to reach chosen targets involve gathering and analysis of pertinent information. Marketing information systems become a vital part of marketing management. Collection of information, analyses of information and continuous monitoring of market behavior becomes an integral part of marketing management activities.

Segmentation

... [T]he first task in formulating a marketing strategy is to select market targets, that is, selection of particular groups of customers or a segment of the market. Thus a market itself is nothing but a sum of these segments. In this context, target means a particular segment or segments that the organization wishes to serve. Choice of segments is based on the organization's resources, products, location and "fit" with the needs of consumers. Selection of target segments imply that the organization makes a choice from among several segments and also a choice based on those segments offering greatest return at appropriate risks. Business firms have come to segment their markets because of the realization that catering to all the segments of a market is neither prudent management policy nor profitable in the long run. So they attempt to find their "best fit" (niche) and design the marketing mix to suit their unique segments.

Consumer Analysis—Marketing and Health Care

The analysis of segments necessarily involves consumers and their needs. Therefore, consumer analysis—their perceptions, needs and behavior—becomes an integral first step before any determination of segments is made. Consumer analyses involve the purchase and usage behavior of present and potential consumers, their demographic and other characteristics, psychological variables and the like. It also involves the analysis of consumer decision making processes with respect to different products and services. In the health services area, Rosenstock[1] has found that the consumers' psychological state of readiness to take specific actions depends on the perception of consumers on their susceptibility, their perception of how serious the health problem is and their perception of benefits of taking such actions. Other analyses use variations of this basic model. This is not unlike the models in consumer behavior with respect to product purchases, where the consumers; perceptions of the benefits to be derived from a purchase and their perception of risk in that purchase are taken into account in the consumer analysis stage. Consumer intentions (similar to the readiness to act stage of Rosenstock) act as proxy for actual purchase behavior. Just as differing segments exist for a variety of consumer products, there are differing segments for prevention. For example, differences in their needs for prevention may obviously vary with age, sex, education and income. Certain age groups are more likely to be at risk with respect to certain diseases. Suffice it to point out that identification of target segments for different services in the prevention area is possible to ascertain the needs, perceptions and related information from consumers.

Marketing Planning Considerations

Planning of the marketing mix and decisions regarding which elements will be combined in what way, also constitute an integral part of marketing strategy. The four elements—product, price, promotion (communication) and place—can be combined in a variety of ways and coordinated into a single effort to reach the targets. Even if one works with only 10 variations in each of these four elements, there would be 10,000 possible combinations. In addition, marketing mix decisions also involve considerations of all the elements simultaneously. Also, any program of marketing mix variables chosen and implemented must be continuously monitored and changed so as to be adaptable to the dynamism of the market place.

While marketing mix considerations and their formulations are beyond the scope of this introductory paper, several areas of application can briefly be sketched here. For example, business firms attempt to assess the "fit" of the potential product offering by engaging in testing at various stages before a product is introduced. Concept testing procedures are employed to evaluate the accessibility of the concept to consumers and progress through prototype testing, test marketing and finally market introduction of the product. In addition, during these testing stages, information regarding the type of attributes desired by consumers, and the benefits expected to be derived by them are obtained. Such information enables the designing of the configuration of product attributes that is more likely to be successful. Consumers' perceptions of other existing products and services, their positioning in the market all help to "position" the products for the relevant segments. Considerable research time is also spent in arriving at a name, packaging and other elements related to the product. These useful techniques are applicable to arrive at a proper configuration of preventive health care services to be offered to consumers.

In the communication (promotion) area, there are choices to be made regarding allocation of resources between advertising and personal selling and between different media (media mix). Choice of media, time schedules, advertising or selling appeals, themes for advertising campaigns, etc. are all carefully chosen to get the best fit between the media and appeals chosen and the intended target. In addition, promotional schedules are determined taking into account variations in the media schedule and the need for repetition, etc. Also, the effectiveness of promotional mix and promotional efforts are constantly monitored to assure the maximum reach of targeted audience at minimum cost with maximum impact. Such lack of careful and long range planning with respect to promotion of prevention is evident if one looks at the current "educational campaigns" for immunization, drug abuse and other similar measures. Not only are these low budget promotions, but the timing, the fit between the medium and the intended audience etc. need considerable improvement. Such activities need to be coordinated with other elements of the marketing mix, which is also lacking in the present campaign for some of the prevention indicated above. For example, the immunization promotion sponsored by indemnity-type insurers exhort consumers to get immunizations for their children, but none of which are reimbursable under most of the present insurance plans (other preventive health care visits also suffer from this lack of coverage).

Pricing as an element of the marketing mix is very useful in introduction of new products or for increasing usage of presently available products etc. In the prevention area, there is no information generally available to potential consumers regarding the pricing for these services. Since the "prices" are fixed by medical societies and the like and no information is available to the general public, the normal pricing policies, such as penetration pricing etc. cannot be availed by preventive health care services marketing at the present time. Such "price fixing" while not permitted in the consumer product arena is already under scrutiny by Federal Trade Commission and other agencies. In the near future, "pricing" as an element of the controllable variables will become available to the prevention area as well. Flexibility in pricing policies, combined with innovative and imaginative incentives to supplement prices will help provide integrated marketing for preventive health care services.

Finally, the logistical aspects of offering preventive health care services at locations convenient and accessible have largely been unrecognized so far. Once the configuration of preventive health care services to be offered are determined, the delivery points and methods can be developed. To make them widely accessible, policies similar to "intensive distribution" of consumer products can be formulated and such preventive services would then become available in as many locations as possible. They may well be offered at supermarkets, at the places of work, shopping centers and may even be available in "franchised" type outlets across the country. Specialized outlets ("boutiques") for specialized preventive health care services (e.g., mammography) can spring up. Increased use of telemetric devices and computerized diagnostic services can result in unique new outlets, particularly in rural areas. Innovative ways to deliver the "product" (prevention) can be developed, if such decisions are coordinated with other elements of the marketing mix.

The concepts, techniques and technologies of marketing research and marketing management are already available. We also have abundant experience with their use for products and services. What is needed now is a recognition that such marketing management practices are applicable to preventive health care area and make creative modifications to adapt them to special nature of prevention. The immediate marketing problem is to make the segments at risk "users" of preventive health care services. Then the problem of making them "repeat customers" emerges.

PROBLEMS OF IMPLEMENTATION

While the relevance of the marketing process to the preventive health care area may have become obvious, introducing the concepts and practices of marketing will face difficulties.

The first problem is one of attitude of health care professionals. In their view, it is demeaning to sell health. Hochbaum's observations are characteristic of others in this field:[2]

> . . . it may be said that we are trying to sell people something they really want: health, a long life, and all the goodies that are presumed to be associated with health. But do we need to sell health? Surely, people do want to live a long productive life, free from disease and disability. There can be no doubt that all but a small minority of people do. People are already sold on health. The problem is something else.

Contrary to what physicians and health care professionals view as the "life giving" endeavour that they are engaged in, the typical consumer seems to consider all health care expenditures in relation to other expenditures for food, clothing and shelter. More importantly just as business firms usually reduce the expenditure for preventive health services as amenable for cuts during their budget crunch.

The second problem is one of ethical considerations. Health care professionals are genuinely concerned about what price-competition and advertising will do to the quality of health care and dignity of the profession. It is ironic that health care providers who operate and depend on the market place for their survival, have very little faith in the competitive system. If professionals will tamper with the quality because of advertising or disclosure of price and price-competition, then the problem lies with their value system and their training. However, the concerns expressed are valid and such objections can be overcome if it can perhaps be regulated as a service industry, similar to airlines as an example.

The third problem stems from the unrealistic expectations and unattainable standards that are professed for evaluating the success of any prevention program. The argument is that the criteria by which success are evaluated in the commercial area cannot be applied to the preventive health arena. Hochbaum[2] makes the following argument that many in this area make:

> Consider a hypothetical manufacturing company whose product is bought by, say, 20 percent of its potential consumer population. If a sales campaign succeeded in increasing this volume by another five percent in one year, the company would probably be highly pleased. But if a health program that tried to get all women at risk of cervical cancer to have a

yearly pap smear, attracted only 20 or even 30 or 40 percent to begin with and succeeded only to add another five or ten percent to this number, the program would be regarded as a failure. Indeed, what would be proudly proclaimed as victory in the commercial arena, will often be bemoaned as defeat in the health arena.

One needs not have to be reminded that "Rome was not built in a day," nor can we ignore the slow increase in seeking prevention from the most risk prone segments. Slow growth is preferable to not attempting to reach them in the high expectation of holding out for 100% participation (usage rate).

Conclusion

In concluding, it is reasonable to argue that the problems that are apparent in the implementation stage of marketing practices are not at all that insurmountable. After all, both the health professional and the marketing practitioner are interested in the same goal in the prevention health measures. If marketing activities are likely to induce greater participation by the very segments which need prevention, then application of marketing techniques to promote physician-generated prevention are worth a try.

REFERENCES

1. Rosenstock, Irwin M. "Why People Use Health Services," *Milbank Memorial Fund Quarterly,* Vol. 44 (July 1966), pp. 94–127.

2. Hochbaum, Godfrey M. "Selling Health to the Public," in *Consumer Behavior in the Health Marketplace.* Editor: Ian M. Newman, Nebraska Center for Health Education, University of Nebraska, Lincoln, Nebraska, pp. 5–14.

29. The Marketing Audit: A Tool for Health Service Organizations

ERIC N. BERKOWITZ AND WILLIAM A. FLEXNER

Reprinted from *Health Care Management Review*, Vol. 3, no. 4, Fall 1978, by permission of Aspen Systems Corporation, © 1978.

Recent articles have explained the philosophy of marketing health services. Highlighted here are the important concerns in the "hands-on" development and implementation of a marketing plan.

Marketing is increasingly recognized as an effective tool in the management of health services. Some potential benefits recently cited in the literature include: improved capacity to respond to the needs and wants of consumers, personnel and the community in general; clarification in the development of long-range strategies and objectives; and more effective allocation of resources within the organization.[1-3]

Marketing of health services involves analyzing organizational interactions (transactions) with donors, patients, employees and regulators of the organization.[4] However, before undertaking any marketing program, the factors that affect the organization's internal operations and its relations with the environment must be assessed. As Ireland notes:[5]

> Ideally, a hospital that is developing a marketing program should begin by conducting a series of research studies to gather information that will help define the characteristics, needs, and wants of its market and marketing segments, so that it can develop or revise its services and accommodations accordingly.

Unfortunately, assessments such as Ireland proposes are often done late in the planning process of health organizations. However, an early marketing inquiry—the marketing audit—may be more beneficial.

NOTE: The authors thank Steven R. Orr, Vice President, Corporate Planning, Fairview Community Hospitals, Minneapolis, Minnesota, for his assistance in the preparation of this article.

TWO APPROACHES TO PLANNING

Typically, the planning sequence in health organizations includes the specification of goals, translation of these into operational objectives, development of strategies to achieve the goals and objectives, implementation of the strategies, and finally feedback or evaluation to modify or adjust current strategies and implementation procedures.[6] Figure 1 shows this sequential process.

In this planning approach, understanding the organization's environment and particularly its marketplace usually occurs after the product and service strategies have been defined. While this information may aid in "selling" the product or services being offered, the timing is too late to determine whether the products or services being produced are those that are wanted or needed.

Marketing literature and practice provide another planning sequence. (See Figure 2.) In this model, the consumer of health services (whether viewed as the physician, the patient, the government or some other purchaser) is recognized as the focal point for making the key choices that dictate the organization's success. With a marketing approach, the consumer is considered at the beginning of the planning process.[7] Consumers may be grouped into segments based on behavior or needs. Included in this initial analysis are a consideration of both

Figure 1 A Typical Health Planning Model

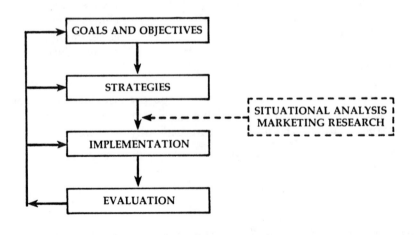

Figure 2 A Marketing Planning Model

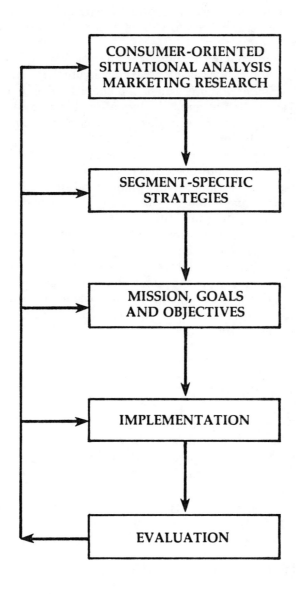

the internal capabilities of the organization, and the preferences and needs of the organization's current and potential consumers. This examination of the organization's internal aspects identifies the range of activities that can be performed, as well as the strong and weak points among these activities.

Once this situational or segmentation analysis is completed, the second step in the process associates various strategies with particular segments of consumers. Forecasts of the potential demand from each segment are then often attempted. Only after this step has been completed does the organization consider specific goals and objectives, and the means for implementing the chosen strategies.

As can be seen, the two approaches differ only in terms of the process flow. This difference, however, is critical in terms of structuring consumer-responsive strategies and plans. Traditionally, health service organizations have planned from the inside to the consumer. Yet regulatory, resource and competition trends are requiring the change from a traditional to a marketing planning strategy. A marketing approach starts the process with the consumer, letting the consumer's needs and wants guide the strategy of the organization. Here the consumer is at the beginning of the planning process, around which selective strategies, objectives and goals are constructed. For any organization changing to a marketing orientation, the process should begin with a marketing audit.

THE MARKETING AUDIT

Audits have typically been a procedure used in accounting for internal control. Because marketing can be a critical activity contributing to the efficient and effective operation of any organization, the need for marketing audits in nontraditional businesses is increasing. As many health organizations begin to recognize the marketing function and to formulate marketing objectives, an early marketing audit is essential. This process provides a foundation on which to develop programs and standards for evaluation.

The Meaning of a Marketing Audit

In its most basic sense, an audit is an evaluation of a firm's activities. Bell has suggested that "a marketing audit is a systematic and thorough examination of a company's marketing position."[8] Shuchman more precisely outlines this practice as:[9]

... a systematic, critical, and impartial review and appraisal of the total marketing operation: of the basic objectives and policies and the assumptions which underlie them as well as the methods, procedures, personnel, and organization employed to implement the policies and achieve the objectives.

A variety of reasons for conducting a marketing audit exists. The dynamic nature of society and the health care industry, in particular, requires up-to-date information for the organization to operate effectively. One must periodically monitor the organization's position and activities to assess their responsiveness to market needs and preferences.

In this dynamic environment, a marketing audit has many purposes:[10]

- It appraises the total marketing operation.
- It centers on the evaluation of objectives and policies and the assumptions that underlie them.
- It aims for prognosis as well as diagnosis.
- It searches for opportunities and means for exploiting them as well as for weaknesses and means for their elimination.
- It practices preventive as well as curative marketing practices.

The Nature of an Audit

Conducting an audit can be an extremely complex task. In essence, it involves examining the entire scope of the organization's activities. Through a broad-based approach, certain cogent issues within each area of marketing operations (product and service design, promotion, price, location) can be identified for analysis in greater depth. Figure 3 shows the scope of the marketing audit procedure.

The audit process is represented as a series of circles expanding outward from the consumer. One begins by looking at the size of the consumer market and the various ways that it can be divided or segmented. To this information must be added information concerning one's own health service organization. Often there are internal constraints that must be determined before devising marketing strategies. Beyond the organization, an assessment needs to be made of the competition, its strengths and weaknesses.

Cutting across each of these circles are the organizing or controllable variables that ultimately come together to define the marketing strategy. These marketing mix variables include the product or service offered, the price at which it is offered, the way in which it is promoted

Figure 3 The Scope of the Marketing Audit

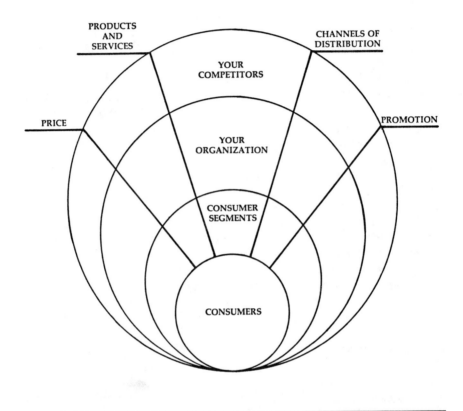

and the channels through which the product or service is distributed.[11] At each stage of the marketing audit, these variables must be considered.

Areas of Inquiry in the Marketing Audit Procedure

For any organization, some factors may appear more relevant than others. The more important and common areas of inquiry for each circle represented in Figure 3 will be listed here in the form of questions to serve as a guide in the marketing audit process. These questions indicate that an audit is an information gathering process. Analysis will then depend on the audit team's foresight and management skill.

THE MARKET AND MARKET SEGMENTS

- How large is the territory covered by your market? How have you determined this?
- How is your market grouped?
  - Is it scattered?
  - How many important segments are there?
  - How are these segments determined (demographics, service usage, attitudinally)?
- Is the market entirely urban, or is a fair proportion of it rural?
- What percentage of your market uses third party payment?
  - What are the attitudes and operations of third parties?
  - Are they all equally profitable?
- What are the effects of the following factors on your market?
  - Age
  - Income
  - Occupation
  - Increasing population
  -
  - Decreasing birthrate } demographic shifting
- What proportion of potential customers are familiar with your organization, services, programs?
  - What is your image in the marketplace?
  - What are the important components of your image?

THE ORGANIZATION

- Short history of your organization:
  - When and how was it organized?
  - What has been the nature of its growth?
  - How fast and far have its markets expanded? Where do your patients come from geographically?
  - What is the basic policy of the organization? Is it on "health care," "profit"?
  - What has been the financial history of the organization?
    - How has it been capitalized?
    - Have there been any account receivable problems?
    - What is inventory investment?
  - What has been the organization's success with the various services promoted?
- How does your organization compare with the industry?
  - Is the total volume (gross revenue, utilization) increasing, decreasing?
  - Have there been any fluctuations in revenue? If so, what were they due to?
- What are the objectives and goals of the organization? How can they be expressed beyond the provision of "good health care"?

- What are the organization's present strengths and weaknesses in:
  - Medical facilities
  - Management capabilities
  - Medical staff
  - Technical facilities
  - Reputation
  - Financial capabilities
  - Image
- What is the labor environment for your organization?
  - For medical staff (nurses, physicians, etc.)?
  - For support personnel?
- How dependent is your organization upon conditions of other industries (third party payers)?
- Are weaknesses being compensated for and strengths being used? How?
- How are the following areas of your marketing function organized?
  - Structure
  - Manpower
  - Reporting relationships
  - Decision-making power
- What kinds of external controls affect your organization?
  - Local?
  - State?
  - Federal?
  - Self-regulatory?
- What are the trends in recent regulatory rulings?

COMPETITORS

- How many competitors are in your industry?
  - How do you define your competitors?
  - Has this number increased or decreased in the last four years?
- Is competition on a price or nonprice basis?
- What are the choices afforded patients?
  - In services?
  - In payment?
- What is your position in the market—size and strength—relative to competitors?

PRODUCTS AND SERVICES

- Complete a list of your organization's products and services, both present and proposed.
- What are the general outstanding characteristics of each product or service?
- What superiority or distinctiveness of products or services do you have, as compared with competing organizations?
- What is the total cost per service (in-use)? Is service over/under utilized?
- What services are most heavily used? Why?
  - What is the profile of patients/physicians who use the services?
  - Are there distinct groups of users?

Continued on next page

The marketing audit is the starting point. Examining the issues raised in these questions will allow a more viable, effective marketing strategy to be developed. For the health organization beginning its marketing plan, the audit process will establish parameters for the program and goals to be accomplished.

Many of the questions raised within the marketing audit already are being considered in some form by health planners. In this sense, mar-

- What are your organization's policies regarding:
  — Number and types of services to offer?
  — Assessing needs for service addition/deletion?
- History of products and services (complete for major products and services):
  — How many did the organization originally have?
  — How many have been added or dropped?
  — What important changes have taken place in services during the last ten years?
  — Has demand for the services increased or decreased?
  — What are the most common complaints against the service?
  — What services could be added to your organization that would make it more attractive to patients, medical staff, nonmedical personnel?
  — What are the strongest points of your services to patients, medical staff, nonmedical personnel?
  — Have you any other features that individualize your service or give you an advantage over competitors?

PRICE

- What is the pricing strategy of the organization?
  — Cost-plus
  — Return on investment
  — Stabilization
- How are prices for services determined?
  — How often are prices reviewed?
  — What factors contribute to price increase/decrease?
- What have been the price trends for the past five years?
- How are your pricing policies viewed by:
  — Patients
  — Physicians
  — Third party payers
  — Competitors
  — Regulators

PROMOTION

- What is the purpose of the organization's present promotional activities (including advertising)?
  — Protective
  — Educational
  — Search out new markets
  — Develop all markets
  — Establish a new service
- Has this purpose undergone any change in recent years?
- To whom has advertising appeal been largely directed?
  — Donors
  — Patients
    — Former or current
    — Prospective
  — Physicians
    — On staff
    — Potential
- What media have been used?
- Are the media still effective in reaching the intended audience?
- What copy appeals have been notable in terms of response?
- What methods have been used for measuring advertising effectiveness?
- What is the role of public relations?
  — Is it a separate function/department?
  — What is the scope of responsibilities?

CHANNELS OF DISTRIBUTION

- What are the trends in distribution in the industry?
  — What services are being performed on an outpatient basis?
  — What services are being provided on an at-home basis?
  — Are satellite facilities being used?
- What factors are considered in location decisions? When did you last evaluate present location?
- What distributors do you deal with? (e.g., medical supply houses, etc.)
- How large an inventory must you carry?

keting planning may seem no different from methods presently used. Yet the key difference is *when* these questions are examined. A marketing orientation begins with the consumers of the service. The audit process then continues internally after information is gained from the market place. This approach follows an external sequence, while traditional health planning methods proceed in the opposite direction.

Because the health care organization operates in a dynamic environment, the audit should become a part of the regular planning sequence. Each question should be reevaluated to highlight changes that may have important strategic implications for the organization in fulfilling its goals.

The marketing audit provides guidance for improving the organization's profitability, competitive position and overall performance. This is accomplished by clarifying the setting in which strategies, goals and objectives related to future action can be intelligently generated.

REFERENCES

1. Ireland, R. C. "Using Marketing Strategies to Put Hospitals on Target."*Hospitals* 51 (June 1, 1977) p. 54–58.

2. O'Halloran, R. D., Staples, J. and Chiampa, P. "Marketing Your Hospital." *Hospital Progress* 57 (1976) p. 68–71.

3. Clarke, R. N. "Marketing Health Care: Problems in Implementation." *Health Care Management Review* 3:1 (Winter 1978) p. 21–27.

4. Shapiro, B. P. "Marketing for Nonprofit Organizations." *Harvard Business Review* (September-October 1973) p. 123–132.

5. Ireland. "Using Marketing Strategies." p. 55.

6. Hyman, H. *Health Planning* (Germantown, Md.: Aspen Systems Corporation 1975) Ch. 3.

7. Keith, R. J. "The Marketing Revolution." *Journal of Marketing* (January 1960) p. 35–38.

8. Bell, M. L. *Marketing: Concepts and Strategies* 2nd ed. (Boston: Houghton Mifflin Co. 1972) p. 428.

9. Shuchman, A. "The Marketing Audit: Its Nature, Purposes, and Problems," in *Analyzing and Improving Marketing Performance, Report No. 32* (New York: American Management Association, 1959) p. 13.

10. Shuchman. "The Marketing Audit." p. 15.

11. McCarthy, E. J. *Basic Marketing: A Managerial Approach* 5th ed. (Homewood, Ill.: Richard D. Irwin, Inc. 1975).

30. Marketing: A New Opportunity for Hospital Management

RICHARD C. IRELAND

Adapted by the author from an article originally published in *Hospitals, Journal of the American Hospital Association*, Volume 51, June 1, 1977, copyright 1977, American Hospital Association.

The key to the success, present and future, of any organization, and hospitals particularly, lies, in part, in its ability to accurately and continously assess the needs of the various groups of people it opts to serve and the marketing opportunities available.

For hospitals the rush to attract physician, employee, patient and donor markets, to name a few, is on. And the competition is growing intense. But the race is not likely to be won only by those institutions that are, at the present time, large and financially strong. While size and fiscal health are real assets, another element is necessary. Those hospitals most likely to thrive in the future are those who recognize that the needs, interests, and expectations of the people in their trade area are central to their success.

Certainly any administrator would say that the purpose of his or her hospital is to provide high quality health care to the people in their trade area. Such a statement certainly implies a marketing orientation. However, hospitals have until the last five years, approached the market place from an inside-out orientation. That is, they have developed services without the benefit of good market research. The "inside-out approach" tends to work in a sellers market. Today, however, hospitals are increasingly finding themselves in a buyers market which requires an "outside-in approach". So rather than developing a service based on assumptions, the "outside-in" approach demands that the needs, interests, expectations and willingness to consume, of the hospital's various constituencies be precisely determined *before* the service is established.

This is not meant to imply that hospitals are not serving their various constituencies. Most are. It means that most are doing so without the benefit of an organized marketing program. Many hospitals simply react to markets they happen to find themselves in rather than taking the initiative to serve markets of their own choosing.

Many argue that hospitals have, in fact, been practicing marketing for years. Maybe. It is certainly true that nearly everyone: individuals, groups, organizations engage in marketing activities, e.g., personal selling, advertising, public relations, publications, sales promotion, every day. But few practice the marketing concept. So when it is said that hospitals have been practicing marketing for a long time, what is really meant is that they have been using marketing activities. Moreover, even though these basic marketing tools have been used for decades, there is seldom a coordinated program. The focus of a marketing system is on the overall management of a hospital's marketing activities in order to produce a predetermined set of outcomes.

The primary purpose of a marketing program is to direct the purpose and resources of the hospital toward the needs, interests, and expectations of people in the various markets it opts to serve. And the first clue to developing a successful marketing program is to place the responsibility for the entire marketing program under the management of a high level administrator.

The core concept of marketing is the notion of exchange. Exchange has been around since there were more than two people present on the earth. It has evolved from simple bartering and often coercion, into a mature principle of want satisfaction. To understand the meaning and process of exchange is to understand the essence of marketing. The basis for exchange depends on the answers that a hospital gives to the questions: What are we really selling? What is our customer (physician, patient, employee, and so on) really buying? Very often the answers are not the same. They should be. And, if your hospital is doing an effective job of marketing, they will be! How is it possible for a client to be buying one thing and a hospital to be selling another? It happens all the time. The clue lies in the word, really—what are you *really* selling? Hospitals, as well as many other organizations, often tend to view their mission too narrowly: they may be providing sick care when they should be providing health care. Colleges, for example, no longer are in the business of selling access to knowledge, or job skills, though many still claim they are. The ones that are in the market are selling careers! The task of the hospital marketer, therefore, is to manage exchange activities. Marketing is a hot number on the agendas of many hospital administrators. It should be ! A well organized marketing program can offer a fresh approach to the many problems that hospitals are facing. But many administrators are looking to marketing in the hopes of solving occupancy problems. To develop a marketing program to solve occupancy problems is the wrong approach to marketing. A hospital will solve its occupancy problems because it has an effective marketing program!

There is no question that hospitals need to achieve a deeper understanding of their markets: (physicians, patients, employees, business/ industry, other providers, donors, special interest groups and the community), if they are to keep up with the competition, allocate resources effectively, and to develop the kinds of services each of their various markets need, want, and are willing to utilize. It is also crucial that hospitals build stronger relationships with community markets. Typically, health care services are sought only when the need is curative in nature. Patients, in other words, do not seek services from a hospital, or physician, unless they are experiencing some type of atypical discomfort or have an obvious health problem. Therefore, a hospital is able to respond only to the initiative of the patient. And, to top it off, patients typically know very little about the health care system and often make. their choices haphazardly. A well organized, managed, marketing program, supported by top management; can make a significant contribution to developing the type of health care services that people need. By building awareness and support for that hospital, if a health care need arises (curative or preventative) that "well organized" institution will most likely be the "hospital of choice."

MARKETING IN THE PROFIT SECTOR

The marketing concept was formally developed in the profit sector in the early fifties and credited by some authorities to General Electric. The emphasis was on what the consumer needed not on what General Electric wanted to sell. This development may have been the beginning of the "marketing generation" in American business. And while many businesses are increasingly involved in marketing, the overall orientation in business is toward selling. So while it may be tempting to look to the profit sector for guidance in marketing, the actual resources may be limited.

Marketing in a hospital may be a far more complicated process than is likely to be found in most businesses. For example, a hospital is totally dependent on an outside agent (the physician) over which it has little direct control. Furthermore, the delivery of services are carefully scrutinized and the basis for utilization examined thoroughly. In the business sector, the airlines, for example, could care less whether a trip is justified. Likewise it is a rare occasion when the consumer is asked if he or she really needs a particular product or service. There is far more emphasis in health care on the value or utility that a patient receives.

Another key difference is the extent to which hospitals rely on formal and informal referral systems. While every successful organization relies on referral, or word of mouth, hospitals are dependent on it. A successful marketing program may alter that, however. The time may come when patients are referred to physicians solely through a hospital rather than through an informal referral system.

And finally, there is probably no other industry that requires as many people to be in direct contact with the customer as does the delivery of health care services. Even in the hotel industry direct contact with hotel personnel is minimal.

THE MARKETING PROGRAM

Because of the range of services a hospital offers, it is inefficient to deal with people as if they were an amorphous mass. Frequently, however, many hospitals approach the market in a diffused manner that treats the whole service as an undifferentiated mass of consumers. A diffused marketing approach is used to create overall awareness and support for the hospital as a place to receive specific health care services. It is a poor strategy for developing utilization of a particular service.

An effective hospital marketing program begins by subdividing, or segmenting, the total trade area into groups of health care consumers who are similar with respect to certain demographic variables, health needs, psychological needs, interests or utilization factors. And the best approach is to identify and serve several segments, or target markets, at once. Identifying members of a market segment is a tough assignment for any hospital marketer. Not only must they be identified, they must be capable of being reached with a communications effort. That is, they must be accessible. And finally, they must be aware of their needs so that they will respond to the hospital's offer.

In any case, each target market that is identified will require a separate marketing strategy. The strategy typically includes four variables, the marketing mix which is represented by the Health Care Marketing C.A.P.S. (described in the introduction to Section IV of this book) or, in the business venacular, the "four Ps": Considerations or costs (price), Accessibility (place), Promotion and Service (product). It is the task of the hospital marketer to influence the target market by manipulating the elements of the marketing mix.

The primary emphasis of the marketing mix is that a marketing program, to be complete, requires that all of the C.A.P.S. be considered. Success in applying the marketing mix to a given target market lies in developing a thorough understanding of the people in that market so that the right product can be offered at the right time in the right place supported by the right promotional effort. Indeed, rightness is a key element in successfully applying the marketing mix concept.

DEVELOPING AN ANALYTICAL STRATEGY

In order to make the right, or best, market mix decisions for a given market segment it is imperative the hospital marketer develop an effective research program that will provide reliable information upon which good mix decisions can be used.

The purpose of research is to delineate the actual and potential consumers, their needs and wants, in a given market segment. A second, and equally important, role for research is to continually assess the pay-off of the hospital's marketing activities. The purpose of research is to provide a steady flow of reliable information about the hospital's markets. The market knowledge that is available to the hospital can provide the basis for a competitive advantage in the hospital's trade area.

The questions that need to be considered in shaping a good research program are: What do we really want to know about this group? What decisions do we need to make? How will we proceed to collect the information?

COSTS OR PRICING AS A MARKETING STRATEGY

Many hospital administrators are waking up to the fact that today's health care consumer is becoming "shopper-oriented" or price sensitive. While this always has been the case in maternity services, people are shopping around more. This will become even more apparent as people switch to deductible health insurance. And research shows that health insurance costs are one of the primary concerns of most employees. This is a significant change given the fact that traditionally research has shown that the health care consumer is not, because of insurance coverage, price sensitive.

Pricing given the constraints of Medicare regulations, rate review commissions, and other third party pressures, is not as flexible a variable as it is for a business enterprise. Many businesses, particularly the retail industry, manipulate price, through regular sales and discount, as a major part of their marketing strategy. For the most part, a business can, within the limits of antitrust regulations, charge what the market will bear.

Pricing, as a marketing variable, includes more than the dollar cost of a service. It includes transportation, parking, time off from work, and convenience of payment. Accepting credit cards for payment is basically a pricing decision and may contribute significantly to the decision to use the hospital; particularly the emergency room.

While the effect of a hospital's pricing structure on demand for restorative or curative services is basically insensitive, it is probably an important factor in the demand for elective, nonserious services like cosmetic surgery, screening tests, stress testing, educational programs and certain patient services that relate mostly to comfort. So pricing strategy can be a significant factor for those services not covered by insuranc..

Demand for noncurative services is also related to the knowledge the consumer has about the value, or benefits of a service the more likely it is that they will be willing to pay the price. So the effect of price upon demand is also a function of how well the hospital communicates the value of its services to its markets.

ACCESSIBILITY: FIND THE RIGHT PLACE

In a classic marketing sense, place refers to the timely distribution of goods and services through channels, wholesale outlets, and sales agents, so that products are efficiently delivered to the market place. From a business perspective, place decisions are made in terms of outlets, warehousing, transportation routes, satellite production facilities and access to raw materials. Making the right place decisions is crucial to both business and health care.

The term used for place in health care is access to services. Access refers to the hours the hospital admitting office is open, the 24 hour emergency and pharmacy service, the surgery schedule, the appointment only policy of the x-ray department, the hours the food service is open, the signs (not always easy to find) that direct people to various locations in the hospital, the distance and travel time from the physician's office to the hospital, and the proximity of one department to another.

Accordingly, in planning its service mix for a target market, a hospital needs to consider the following questions in order to determine the right access strategy: How far is the hospital from major physician concentrations? Is the service scheduled at times convenient for physician and patients? How long does it take for patients to get to the service location? Do patients know how to find the service location? Should variations of the service be made available? Is parking adequate? Are admitting and scheduling procedures adequate? Is information about the service or hospital readily available?

Access is the critical linkage of the hospital and relationships through which services are efficiently delivered to consumers desiring or needing an exchange relationship with the hospital. A carefully planned access strategy formulated on reliable market information can significantly improve service utilization by providing needed health care services at a place most accessible to the consumer.

Home health care programs, multi-speciality clinics, mobile health vans, "meals on wheels", the physicians office annex, visiting nurse programs, emergency helicopter services, community-based health education programs, telemetry, phone access to health information, and industrial medical clinics; are all good examples of decisions to offer better access to much needed services. Unfortunately, many access decisions are not based on good marketing research. They should be! If they were, there would be fewer failures.

PROMOTING YOUR SERVICE

After the needs of the consumer by market segment have been determined, the right service mix developed, the price structure established, and the access strategy implemented, an important, and often difficult part of the marketing mix needs to be developed. Prospective consumers must be made aware that the service exists. They have to be persuaded that the service has the desired set of attributes. The information and appeals to be disseminated must be based on a solid understanding the consumers need to know and the various communication channels that the consumer has access to.

Promotion generally refers to advertising, personal selling, public relations, and various incentives. However, the hospital public relations function is often forced to be responsible for many of the classic market promotion activities in a hospital.

For business, selling and advertising are the most commonly used promotional tools. Selling assumes that the prospective customer is most likely to buy when approached by a trained salesperson with an organized presentation. There are degrees of selling and everyone, in every organization, is involved in selling all of the time. In a hospital selling takes place when a prospective donor is asked for a contribution, when the administrator asks a business person to sit on the board, when the public relations director trys to interest a reporter in a hot story, or when someone takes a group on a tour of the hospital. This type of approach is often termed as "soft" or "missionary selling." While this form of selling is important, it is unlikely that a hospital will ever need an organized sales force.

All too frequently, hospital marketing communications (a more meaningful term for hospital marketers) are developed without a clear understanding of the market place. Many times the publications program is described as the marketing program! When a hospital sends out messages to the market place without a clear understanding of who is in the market, it risks developing a distorted or fragmented image of itself. Such communication efforts are usually a waste of everyone's time and the hospital's money.

A well defined marketing communications program takes into account the specific information needs of the target market for whom the communications element is intended. The information is valued, usable, accurate, motivating and is developed in a way that facilitates action. In other words the audience understands what it is that the element is trying to do as a result of receiving the message. Communication elements, e.g., publications, news releases, are most effective when they are a part of a complete hospital marketing program. Failure to properly coordinate the communications program is a weakness in many hospitals and one, ironically, that the hospital marketer has the most control over.

In today's health care market there is keen competition for the attention of the consumer, on all fronts. The key task is to attract and retain the attention of an audience in order to make an appeal or deliver a message—and to do it in such a way that the message is understood as intended.

An effective hospital communicator must be thoroughly familiar with the needs and problems of the audience, the message to be communicated and the various techniques and channels that can be most effectively used to reach an audience. When this happens, the communicator becomes a marketer. And too, the hospital marketer must remember that people are attracted to attributes, or benefits, not the service or hospital per se.

SERVICE DEVELOPMENT

On the basis of good market research a hospital selects, or develops, the most appropriate services to be offered a particular market segment. In developing a service it is crucial to realize that an individual doesn't buy a service per se. Rather, what a person really buys is a set of benefits, or attributes. A person is far more interested in what he or she gets out of the service personally rather than its technical dimensions or qualities. And in the end, it is the attributes of the hospital or service that are evaluated, not the hospital or service per se.

An attribute, or benefit, is that aspect of a service that will fulfill a need. Every person has a preference for certain attributes that he or she considers desirable. A service and hospital are favored to the extent that a person believes that certain attributes are present. Therefore, becoming "hospital of choice" is based on the salience of the number of desirable attributes that are present and known to the individual, or target market.

Therefore, to develop demand for a hospital, or service (particularly non-curative services) it is necessary to determine the attributes that are valued by the prospective consumer and then develop the service accordingly. In other words, to be successful in the health care market place a hospital has to put a lot of "sizzle" in its service. And many times the attributes most desired by the consumer are not those that are essential to the service.

The general attributes that a hospital's service mix strategy must consider are the "7Cs" of hospital service development. First, the hospital must provide the right level and quality of "Care." Hospital Care refers to technical capability, e.g., up-to-date equipment, modern facilities, good management systems, competent personnel, and so on. The second attribute concerns the delivery of care, "Caring." Caring refers to the empathy, warmth, and compassion that people delivering the care have for the patient. Related to Caring, ranking three and four, are "Comfort" and "Convenience." Comfort takes into consideration hotel amenities like menu selection and food quality, color television, and decorations. Convenience, probably the most valued attribute in America, refers to ease of admitting, preadmission testing, scheduling, parking, visiting hours, children's waiting room, rooming-in, and the hours that a service operates. Normally, Convenience attributes are those that reduce the amount of hassle a patient has to put up with. And Convenience and Comfort attributes vary dramatically by market segment. Fifth on the list, not in order of priority, are the "Curative" attributes, the ability of the hospital or service to help a person get well. The significant Curative attributes that can be gained from a hospital service are those that are lifesaving in character. The sixth service attribute is one that will help patients "Cope" with their illness or injury. Patient education and therapy are Coping attributes. And finally, the seventh service attribute that nearly everyone has an opinion about is "Cost." Cost attributes are present in the development of day surgery and alternative birthing programs, home care, and the efficiency of the business office.

Service attributes do not generally exist in isolation but are interactive. Comfort, for example, is contingent upon cost, convenience and caring. The point is that when service attributes are selected to meet the needs of a given group of people they combine to produce a synergistic effect. That's marketing!

Finally, it is important that hospital marketers develop a comprehensive inventory of the services being offered by their hospital and other providers. The inventory should include costs, utilization, attributes, demand and market segment served. Normally, an area service inventory, by provider, is part of the area health system plan.

GETTING THE PROGRAM STARTED

An effective marketing program begins with an analysis of where the hospital has been, where it is at the present time, where it wants to go, and, most importantly, a sincere and genuine commitment from the hospital's administration to invest the required resources in the marketing effort. Viewing marketing as an investment with a specified return will help to build needed support and optimize the ability of the hospital to respond effectively to the various needs of its target markets.

Putting together a marketing program should begin by conducting an extensive marketing feasibility audit. The purpose of the audit is to evaluate the extent to which a marketing program is feasible, the hospital's readiness to launch a program, the limitations, if any, and suggestions as to the best place to begin.

The audit is based on the rationale that the most likely and accurate predictor of what is going to happen in the future is a knowledge of what is going on at the present time. An historical analysis is helpful and much can be learned regarding past trends. However, it is the current knowledge, management style, attitude and support, and resources that a hospital will use to embark on its marketing program. Therefore, it is the "right-now" of the hospital situation that will provide the best clues as to what is most likely to happen in the future—regardless of the verbal optimism expressed for a marketing program.

Specifically, the marketing feasibility audit is a comprehensive, internal evaluation of a hospital's current marketing activities, or program. The purpose is to determine the extent that marketing functions are integrated. The audit attempts to review the assumption, conceptions and expectations that guide hospital administrators in their planning and operation decisions. It reviews how people—department directors, medical staff, supervisors—feel about their hospital with respect to the markets they serve.

The underlying assumption of the marketing audit is that the hospital desires to improve the performance of its marketing activities. The focus is on the various ways that the hospital is currently managing those activities. The audit includes a careful examination of the setting the hospital is operating in, an overall evaluation of the hospital's current marketing system, the marketing information system and an evaluation of the communications efforts of the hospital. In addition, an audit, correctly done, will also consider the hospital's current staff capacity for developing a marketing program, the general attitude toward marketing, how proposed and current marketing efforts compare with the competition, and what is currently taking place in terms of utilization.

Hopefully, a completed audit will provide an extensive evaluation on how the hospital utilizes marketing activities and the extent to which it understands and analyzes its trade area. With the commitment of top management and an executed marketing task force under the management of a person who is thoroughly knowledgeable and experienced in implementing the marketing concept. Members of the marketing task force should involve themselves in an extensive interview survey of key individuals, particularly department directors, in the hospital to draw upon their knowledge of the hospital's distinctive competencies and constraints. Such a survey also has a secondary effect of building support and understanding for the marketing program. Politically, it's a sound way to market marketing. In addition to the interview survey, the task force should also conduct an extensive situation analysis that would include an evaluation of the hospital's long range plan and its direct or implied mandates for marketing program. Many times the long range plan objectives are market oriented. A situation analysis would also include an historical audit of records to determine utilization, patient origins, trends, and medical staff composition. If the hospital has a good planning department, most of the information needed for an historical audit should already have been collected.

After the task force has completed its situation analysis, it is in a good position to prepare a preliminary report to the administration that includes their recommendations on how to proceed with the development of the marketing program. The next step would be develop a set of research priorities and objectives to make a precise determination of the attitudes and needs of the hospital's major market segments. The market studies that should be included are a complete audit of patient origin and medical staff composition and utilization over the past three to five years; an attitude and needs survey of former patients, physicians, community, employees, and several community groups; institutional positioning studies to determine where the hospital stands on selected attributes (with selected markets) with respect to other health care providers; consensus surveys on the marketable strengths of the hospital; and a competitive evaluation of other providers in the hospital's trade area.

The next step is to analyze the research results and outline potential markets, draw up objectives and outline a marketing strategy. Priorities should then be assigned to specific market segments and a market mix test formulated for one or two markets of high priority.

Finally, the task force should develop a complete annual marketing plan with policies, objectives, strategies, marketing activities, priorities and schedules, organization and assignments, budgets and allocation of resources, and feedback and review procedures.

SUMMARY

In summary, the basics of a good hospital marketing program are to make a precise determination of what the consumer's needs are. Devise strategies to make them aware of their needs. Develop a service mix that will best meet those needs. Develop a comprehensive communications program that will let them know what the hospital has to offer. Deliver the service with high quality performance. And provide a careful evaluation.

Marketing is relatively new to the hospital industry and to those hospitals wise enough to implement a program, it offers a fresh perspective for securing the hospital's future.

31. The Use of Marketing Strategies in Meeting Changing Needs

DAVID D. KARR

Adapted by the author from an article originally published in *Hospitals, Journal of the American Hospital Association*, Vol. 51, June 1, 1977, copyright 1977, American Hospital Association.

The investor owned hospital companies have brought many changes which have resulted in hospitals approaching management in the same manner as do other industries such as manufacturers of hard goods, fast food chains, and providers of personal services. Principally, the discipline introduced was sound fiscal management which, in its broad interpretation, includes marketing. Marketing in the hospital industry is basically the same as in other industries; that is, it makes the public aware of the services provided, the quality of these services, and, once the services are rendered, takes steps to assure customer satisfaction.

The management of investor-owned companies recognized early in the industry's formative years that little had been done in the area of marketing even though the industry was large and was providing one of the most important basic human needs. It was an industry of little or no competition, depending for the most part on doctors voluntarily joining the medical staff and patients accepting the services they received with little critical evaluation since hospitals were viewed as institutions ranking second only to the church. In many instances, neither the doctors nor the patients had a choice as to the hospital to be used.

The hospital industry has gone through significant changes with the advent of the investor owned multi-hospital companies, the most important being the introduction of competition and consequently the marketing of services. Each of the major multi-hospital companies have well planned marketing programs directed toward increasing both inpatient census and outpatient service volumes.

The initial step in developing a marketing strategy for a hospital is the development of a master business plan. This business plan, used to determine present and future health care needs of the community, includes a detailed profile of the community, demographics, facility usage data and the impact, both negative and positive, of health care laws and of governmental rules and regulations. The business plan should contain five major sections, which are:

1. Service area
2. Population
3. Economic data
4. Professional health manpower availability
5. Statistics on utilization of existing health care facilities

SERVICE AREA

The geographical area served by a hospital is identified through a patient origin study. Changes that may be occurring are identified to determine the rate of change, the timing and the direction of the expected shifts in the service area.

POPULATION

Every detail of population for the service area must be studied including the total number of people, range in ages, the number of people in each age group and local environmental influences on the health of the residents of the service area.

ECONOMIC DATA

The service area must be examined closely to isolate economic influences on health care needs. Primary contributors to the local economy are identified and forecasts made of general economic growth. An analysis of the third party payment sources for health care services should be included in the economic analysis.

PROFESSIONAL HEALTH MANPOWER AVAILABILITY

In addition to determining the number of physicians (by specialty) located in the service area, the study should include the number of nurses and other health care personnel available within the area.

STATISTICS ON UTILIZATION OF EXISTING HEALTH CARE FACILITIES

Data on the community and the hospital are compared to information on other health care facilities. A determination is made as to what illnesses bring local residents to hospitals and which institutions they are using in what numbers. The objective is to find ways to serve current patients better and increase the hospital's share of the base case load.

On completion of the preliminary survey work, marketing directly to the physicians is begun. All hospitals must rely on a strong, active medical staff to achieve high quality patient care, a good rate of utilization, financial strength, and a good reputation. A good insight into physician requirements and ways of filling those requirements to the advantage of the patients is necessary to conduct a successful program.

The Full Service Hospital

A full service institution, operating at a seventy-three percent occupancy rate six months after opening, consistently exceeded 90% the next two and one-half years. A high rate of utilization was forecast from the time of the architect's first drawing. The Regional Planning Agency did not agree with the projections and denied that this hospital was needed. As a result the hospital initially received only token reimbursement from Blue Cross.

The hospital representative worked to turn the situation around quickly. He embarked on a hard-hitting personal selling effort, speaking to civic groups and, more importantly, calling on area physicians. He told the physicians that the hospital offered full surgical capability and provided diagnostic services such as angiographic procedures and isotope studies.

The marketing campaign worked well. Utilization levels shot up, Blue Cross implemented full reimbursement and, finally, the regional planning agency acknowledged the hospital was indeed necessary to the area.

Although the physician is the primary marketing target, work to build goodwill with patients is also important. For example, 15 to 18 percent of this hospital's patients were in the maternity department. It was found that the "Rendezvous Dinner" for new mothers and fathers was a successful marketing tool. More than 30 percent of the maternity patients chose the service. Many reported they came to this hospital expecially because it was offered.

The "Rendezvous Dinner" was also good for staff morale. It gave the dietary department an opportunity to demonstrate their abilities, inasmuch as it featured a gourmet menu with three non-hospital entrees; filet mignon, veal cordon bleu, and flounder stuffed with crabmeat. Prices were consistent with prevailing charges in the area's top quality restaurants. The dinner was served with special china, flatware, nappery and candlesticks. The waiters were fitted with red jackets and received instructions on service of wine. The souvenir menu was printed in good graphic design on fine stock.

The meals were served in quiet areas that had wall to wall carpeting: the solarium, an in-service training room or a small dining room. No more than three couples were served at one time. Placards announcing the service were placed in the maternity area, gift shop and the cafeteria. The marketing message suggested that proud grandparents may wish to purchase the dinner as a gift for the new parents.

On the night of the dinner, a surprise for the patient was added in the form of a complementary bottle of champagne, presented with a gift card attractively engraved by the Company (which owned the hospital) in the name of her obstetrician. This added touch generated goodwill for the corporation with the patient and her doctor.

The Specialty Hospital

At this specialty hospital, which specialized in physical rehabilitation of patients with acute musculoskeletal disorders, marketing efforts worked exceptionally well. The directors of this privately owned facility had a good concept of service when they opened the hospital. They believe in four hours of "hands on" therapy every day for every patient, which was made possible by a high ratio of occupational and physical therapists and physiatrists (sic) to patients.

For the hospital to be successful, the service needed to be promoted to the physicians and health care organizations that could help fill the hospital's beds. For the first six months after the hospital was opened, rarely more than fifty of the eighty available beds were in use at any one time. The hospital's president realized that the management of a major investor owned hospital corporation could help. A management contract was signed with the corporation and the corporate representative put an intensive marketing effort into operation. He started by sending 20,000 pieces of direct mail explaining the hospital's services and the general philosophy behind them to doctors, hospital administrators, continuing care directors and other professionals.

Next, the representative initiated a series of seminars to promote the concept of rehabilitation. The first was a one-day colloquy on sex for the physically disabled. Subsequently, two days were slotted for discussion of an important new form of therapy called proprioceptive neuromuscular facilitation. At a later date, panels of international experts lectured at a six week session of the neurological aspects of rehabilitation. Physicians, nurses, therapists, counselors, psychologists, social workers and administrators from other hospitals attended.

The corporation's representative encouraged media coverage of events at the hospital, and daily newspapers and television and radio stations began allowing space and time for regular discussions of the hospital's activities.

Interest in the hospital burgeoned and the corporate representative zeroed in on a major obstacle to a higher case load: the application form for screening potential patients. It was six pages long and took nine days to process. The representative recommended that a physician's assistant, who is an associate member of the medical staff reporting to the medical director, should meet with patients in their homes or in other hospitals and that they should interview the patients' doctors in order to obtain all information on the original form and more, in a shorter time.

The hospital medical staff agreed, and the corporation's representative was given authority to approve admission within 24 hours for patients whose treatment needs could be satisfied by the hospital's staff and facilities. Further, the referring physician was not required to complete any of the admission forms. The plan put the hospital eight days ahead of others in the area, and once physicians found out they didn't have to fill out forms, the facility experienced a steady increase in its patient census.

Today, the hospital has its full-licensed bed complement in use by patients from all over the United States and from Central and South America who range in age from 15 to 102. Ninety-eight percent of them are referred from general hospitals and the rest come from home or from extended care facilities.

The Expanded Hospital

Sometimes a marketing program is needed to promote greater utilization of a hospital that has been expanded to meet the demands of a growing patient load. Such was the case with a fifty bed hospital built in 1967 on a 15 acre site owned by its medical staff. By 1972, when the hospital was acquired by a multi-hospital chain, the hospital was operating at 100% capacity at all times and was unable to accommodate the growing number of patients seeking its services.

The city had 200,000 residents with an equal number living in its suburbs. The service area clearly needed an expanded health care capability.

The corporation began planning with the hospital's original physician owners, who remained on the staff, to increase the hospital's capacity and to make it a more useful health care resource for the area. Construction was begun on a 105 bed addition which was opened in 1975. The original facility was remodeled for use by short-stay surgical patients, and it reopened in early 1977.

The average length of a patient's stay at the hospital was reduced to 4.06 days, three days below the national average for similar community hospitals. Certain procedures (tonsillectomy, dilation and curettage, and dental surgery) were safely completed, including post operative recuperative time, in 12 hours. A bed in an acute care general hospital need not be occupied for more than a day by patients who have undergone these procedures if they can be transferred safely to their residences or convalescent homes.

The patient was not forced to leave sooner than he or she wished, but all patients were encouraged to take advantage of a shorter time away from home and lower hospital bills, whenever possible. The short stay concept in itself, then, becomes a marketing tool. Patient response, as indicated by the below-average length of stay, was good.

The appeal and practicality of short-stay surgery was combined with pediatric and maternity services, a 10-bed coronary intensive care unit, and the new capabilities of nuclear medicine and cancer treatment. Neither of the area's two other hospitals had a cancer treatment center when planning began, and the hospital then had the most fully equipped oncology unit in the region. In addition to radiation therapy and outpatient chemotherapy, the hospital had the area's only linear accelerator.

The hospital is now a 155 bed institution that no longer operates at a level that tends to restrain the development of good services. The corporation anticipated steadily mounting use and felt the hospital was then fully prepared for a decade of growth in patient census. They have worked to turn the 15 acres on which the hospital is situated into a medical campus. Today, 120 specialists and sub-specialists practice there.

Making new medical services available and attracting physicians to use them is one of investor owned company's strengths. General information is offered on factors that a physician should consider before establishing a practice, such as community development patterns, physician availability, population, relative influence of different health care facilities, mix of health services, presumed need for expansion of or additions to existing services and how community health planning is coordinated.

An Integrated Approach

Good patient and professional relations are the bedrock of a corporation's marketing efforts and should not be separated from other hospital functions. An institution can build and maintain a case load only if all services are functioning as efficient parts of the total hospital health care system. That's where the management engineers fit into the marketing effort. They should analyze all hospital departments through in-depth studies to determine how the quality of patient care can be improved and how operating problems can be resolved. Costs and quality of service must be evaluated to determine the sources of problems. The analysis should include space allocations and equipment, staffing, work loads and work flow. The study will assure the patients of the highest possible efficiency in all aspects of hospital care, including the processing of x-ray, laboratory tests and other diagnostic procedures.

In summary, marketing is the turning of normal hospital activities into advantages. The examples discussed here are but a very few that have worked well. Their success was the result of the free interplay of good ideas between the corporate management and the people in the field, who are the first source of new information on changing service areas.

32. The Emergence of a Marketing Management Approach in a Time of Crisis

DOUGLAS S. SEAVER

Adapted by the author from an article originally published in *Hospitals, Journal of the American Hospital Association*, Vol. 51, June 1, 1977, copyright 1977, American Hospital Association.

June–December 1974: Post Economic Stabilization Program

From June to December 1974, immediately following the Economic Stabilization Program, Methodist Hospital was a troubled institution. It had just avoided bankruptcy, had no capital, and was part of the still unhealthy economy. Furthermore, the hospital would continue to face stringent price controls as third party payors strongly represented their buying publics who remained concerned about hospital costs.

Not only was the experience with the Economic Stabilization Program a concern, but Methodist was beginning to face a serious population shift with concomitant growth of other local hospitals. Three had just undergone expansion. One had moved completely from the inner city of Indianapolis to the northern, well-to-do suburbs.

So, when the hospital inpatient census did not climb back above 80% in the second week of January 1975, following the traditional Christmas decrease, management at Methodist decided it was time to consider shifting its strategy from the restrictive one of cutting expenses to "live within," to an aggressive one of "reaching out." Confronted with that decision Methodist had to answer serious public and institutional questions, but with the end of the Economic Stabilization Program's restrictions also had the freedom to undertake new directions of development.

The public issue was how to make the best use of Methodist Hospital's existing resources, keeping in mind that the population traditionally served was moving away and that hospitals more closely situated to growing population areas were expanding. The answer was to emphasize the hospital's development as a sophisticated referral center. The Board of Trustees decided that Methodist Hospital would become "the private, tertiary care referral center for central Indiana." The recognition that Methodist would be the "private" referral center differentiated it from Indiana University medical school and its hospital. While certain of Methodist's medical services, such as neurosurgery, were drawing patients from all of Indiana, and while certain services, such as obstetrics, would always remain local in focus defining *central* Indiana as the area to be served established a definite market which most services could draw from. The development of strong tertiary care services meant building on a trend which had slowly begun ten years before and aggressively moving the hospital further in that direction.

The institutional dilemma was how to maintain a viable hospital by establishing its tertiary care role and the necessary referral patterns. The answer was to market Methodist Hospital—its image and its services.

However, Methodist Hospital was in the worst possible marketing position. It had virtually no capital, no developmental funds, no usable marketing information. It conducted no continuing marketing research and had no trained or disciplined sales force.

January 1975: Marketing Retreat

It was against this background that on January 20–21, 1975, Methodist Hospital held a marketing retreat: the first time it had seriously broached the idea of going out and selling from Methodist Hospital. Even in the hospital's capital fund raising activities, Methodist had worked through the United Hospital Fund, a consortium of Indianapolis hospitals.

The marketing retreat was a two day affair. The participants included the President of the hospital, the Vice Presidents, the President and other officers of the Medical Staff and directors of the hospital's major revenue producing departments, such as the laboratory, radiology and emergency departments.

Three significant developments resulted from the retreat. First, the developing role of Methodist Hospital as a tertiary referral center was recognized. Potentials for building on this role, emphasizing those sophisticated services in seeking out markets from which to draw referrals, was reinforced as Methodist's basic marketing thrust.

Second, the loose framework of what eventually developed as the hospital's marketing plan emerged. Heretofore, Methodist Hospital had been almost strictly in the "retail business" of selling hospital services through its "salesmen," the medical staff members, to "customers," patients in need of diagnostic and treatment services. Now, Methodist planned to develop a "wholesale market," i.e. other hospitals which would buy services from Methodist and in turn sell them to their own patients. It soon became obvious that the hospital needed a full time marketing director to work with outlying institutions to develop Methodist's "wholesale business."

Third, a long "laundry list" was drawn up with miscellaneous suggestions for better publicity regarding Methodist Hospital's services for new services to be developed, and for suggestions for building Methodist's sales force, i.e. its medical staff.

One of the more unique ideas first explored at the marketing retreat was the development of the admitting department's "outreach" directly into private physician offices. Such outreach would be designed to build rapport with physicians' office staff and to make it as convenient as possible for that physician and his office staff to admit patients to Methodist Hospital. It took about a year for the idea to be fully implemented, but at the present time Methodist Hospital has one full time admitting employee devoted strictly to servicing physicians' offices by going out and explaining the hospital's admissions procedures, providing preadmission information, providing pre-printed physician orders, and the like. This person is a visible representative of Methodist Hospital before its private practicing physicians, so it was important to select such a person carefully.

New programs such as the development of a pediatric pulmonary center to provide a needed service and to shore up the census of the Children's Pavilion (a 112 bed pediatric hospital which is part of Methodist) were agreed on. A suggestion to develop a training program for paramedics who work in county ambulance services was recognized as a way to develop rapport and educate people about Methodist Hospital's services to cultivate potential sources of patients. Also, the idea of a special transport van to carry critically ill newborns to Methodist's Special Care Nursery in the Newborn Center was put forth. Again, this program was one which management felt was sorely needed in the community, but it was also one that offered tremendous visibility and the potential for a lot of publicity through the news media.

The topic of recruiting physicians, particularly certain specialists, was explored. The importance of the hospital's medical education programs, especially its residency programs, was discussed. Medical education builds Methodist's staff directly and increases the number of physicians familiar with Methodist who settle in other parts of Indiana to practice but refer their more complicated cases to their former teachers.

Each of these suggestions and ideas discussed at the marketing retreat, was developed and actually implemented. However, it took the next two years for some of them, for example the pediatric pulmonary center, to appear. Yet the marketing retreat definitely initiated a new focus and perspective for Methodist Hospital.

February–July 1975: Continuing Marketing Discussion

During the next six months, the most important development in the evolution of the concept of marketing at Methodist Hospital was a study written by Marc Voyvodich, the Administrative Resident. The study provided a framework upon which a comprehensive, detailed marketing plan could be designed specifically for Methodist Hospital. It assembled, for the first time for marketing purposes, a tremendous amount of data regarding the services the hospital offered, the markets it served, and the physicians on its medical staff.

The 1975 marketing study concluded with three sets of recommendations: Where to market; what services to market; and how to reach those markets.

Briefly, the emphasis on where to market was two dimensional. First, the study recommended that the hospital market its emergency department services as the strongest way to compete for Marion County patients. Methodist Hospital has the largest and most comprehensive emergency department in the state. Methodist Hospital is the most centrally located hospital in relation to all the major Interstate Highways. Methodist Hospital has the largest and most sophisticated intensive care unit with the capacity to treat the most severely injured patients. These three points, and the fact that the emergency patients contributed heavily to inpatient days, all indicated that the emergency department should be a priority of the hospital's marketing thrust. Hence, the development of the emergency department as a Trauma Center would be undertaken. Also, in another effort to expand the use of the emergency department, the hospital developed specific emergency department links with local industries through such things as direct telephone hook-ups for immediate consultation.

Second, it was recommended that Methodist market inpatient services to other than Marion County patients, emphasizing the development of sophisticated specialty services with specialists located in close proximity to the hospital. Reaching the outlying markets was emphasized as worthwhile because of their expanding population needing to be served and the fact that hospitals in those areas were in the 83-184 bed range. The interstate highway system provides a very convenient access from all of the contiguous counties directly to Methodist.

In terms of what services to market, recommendations emphasized the highly specialized services and deemphasized primary hospital services. It seemed logical to keep patients at their local hospitals whenever possible. This meant not marketing such routine services as obstetrics, even though Methodist had a declining obstetrical volume.

Another issue raised in trying to decide which services to market was whether it was better to build on the hospital's strengths, or shore up its weaknesses. As it turned out, emphasizing and building on its strengths proved to be the more successful approach. The marketing study suggested developing the concept of "centers of excellence" for various medical specialties so that there would be a Methodist Hospital Neurosurgical Center, a Methodist Hospital Cardiovascular Center, and a Methodist Hospital Oncology Center.

In answer to how to reach the markets, the study recommended building rapport with the outlying hospitals through shared service programs as one way to develop the hospital-to-hospital and medical staff-to-medical staff relationship necessary to groom these markets for patient referrals.

September 1975: Computerized Marketing Information System

As an outgrowth of the marketing study, it became clear that the hospital needed to routinely generate patient information to assess the results of the hospital's marketing efforts, and to identify new areas (geographically and by service) for future growth. Management considered it important to have as complete a marketing information system as possible and to be able to track changes in patient volumes on a monthly basis. It was thus decided to design a computerized information system which would collect information from all patients and provide monthly reports. Methodist had a computerized business office system, and the computerized billing tapes which were part of that were selected as an accurate and convenient source of information.

Overall, the system is designed to examine three markets: the hospital's inpatient market, its emergency department market, and its referred outpatient market. To do this five separate reports are generated: 1. a physician utilization report which identifies the volume of business each medical staff member brings to the hospital; 2. an inpatient geographic origin report; 3. a medical service utilization report which notes the number of patients each medical specialty treated at the hospital; 4. an emergency department patient analysis; and 5. an outpatient geographic origin report.

The information from these reports is analyzed, charted, graphed and summarized in a monthly report. The hospital has developed demographic data by zip code so that it knows the average family income, racial composition, etc. per zip code from which it draws patients. As the hospital might undertake new marketing programs such as the sponsorship of a neighborhood health center, the hospital can examine what happens both to outpatient and inpatient utilization from the zip code in which the health center is located. Also, the Indiana Hospital Association and the Former Comprehensive Health Planning Agency provided the number of admissions per 1,000 population by zip code so that Methodist can compare its number of admissions per 1,000 population from any zip code and see what percentage of that market it has captured.

May 1976: Vice President Shared Services

By May of 1976, Methodist Hospital was serious enough about its commitment to marketing that a corporate position of vice president for shared services was created. This position is Methodist Hospital's marketing officer. The title of vice president for shared services, rather than vice president for marketing, was selected because the main thrust of the job is not the "retail marketing" of Methodist to physicians, but the "wholesale marketing" of Methodist's services to other hospitals and health care providers. Creating a full time shared services position was an important decision in the evolution of the concept of marketing at Methodist, for it committed specific manpower to the marketing job and provided a corporate visibility and focus to the hospital's marketing programs.

Because marketing involved selling services to small hospitals in predominantly rural areas, a former administrator of a 100 bed Indiana hospital was selected for the vice president of shared services. The person's entire hospital career had been in small institutions. It was felt that selecting a person who knew the needs of small hospitals, could "talk their language" and who had developed a reputation among hospital administrators of small and rural institutions were important characteristics. In essence, Methodist selected a person for the shared services position based on what it perceived as the ability to relate to that market and sell.

Methodist sells two types of services—administrative services, such as purchasing and management consultation; and clinical services, such as respiratory therapy and clinical pathology. The purpose of selling administrative services is to increase the hospital's revenue through unrelated business income. All such services are priced at full cost plus a net margin. Building new sources of revenue to stabilize the hospital's financial situation is the ultimate goal.

The purpose of selling shared clinical services is twofold: to effect better distribution of scarce health resources within Indiana, and to build the identification hospital-to-hospital and medical staff member-to-medical staff member. It is felt that such an identification will increase referrals, when appropriate, from primary-secondary hospitals to Methodist Hospital as a specialty referral center. Clinical services are priced at full cost only.

A specific example of a shared service program which meets the criteria of keeping patients at their local hospitals, improving the quality of patient care, building rapport with medical staff members and strengthening referral patterns is remote cardiac monitoring by Methodist. The program involves a dedicated telephone hookup with Decatur County Memorial Hospital, a 100 bed institution located 45 miles away. Decatur has a coronary care unit in which patients can be hooked up to cardiac monitors which transmit signals to Methodist Hospital's heart station where 24 hours a day, seven days a week, monitoring is done by specially trained nurses. Internal medicine residents, cardiology fellows and some of the leading cardiologists in the state are available for review and consultation. Computerized electrocardiography is also provided to Decatur Hospital over telephone lines where the computer reads the electrocardiogram which is then overread by a cardiologist and the overreading sent back through the computer and telephone line. EKG scanning equipment is also provided to Decatur County Hospital for use by its attending staff. With the cardiac monitoring program, patients who could not have been kept at Decatur County Hospital, which does not have a cardiologist, now remain there. The quality of patient care is improved by monitoring, and physician rapport is enhanced through consultations. Also, when patients need open heart surgery, the link is established for them to be referred to Methodist Hospital.

December 1976– October 1977: Management Contracts

Two major activities during the initial seven months of Methodist's shared services program involved assessing services needed in small, surrounding hospitals and trying to meet their specific needs.

By the fall of 1976, however, Methodist Hospital had begun to negotiate its first total management contract with a 40-bed community hospital. The first big development in the growing shared services program came about as a direct result of visibility gained through general contacts with outlying institutions.

Methodist Hospital's management contract had two dimensions. First, Methodist agreed to provide a chief executive officer, acceptable to the other hospital's board of trustees, who retains employee status at Methodist as part of its administrative team. This arrangement gave the small hospital an excellent chance to get a "top notch" administrator. In addition, Methodist could offer the administrator continued career opportunities on its staff after two or three years at the community hospital. Second, Methodist Hospital contractually established a consulting fee schedule for input from various department heads and key staff members. Unlike obtaining expertise from consulting firms, these contractual services come from one source and are directly monitored by an administrator responsible to both organizations.

Other contractual arrangements provided continuing medical education, joint purchasing, and physician recruitment services. Methodist Hospital's approach to these areas, outlined in the contract, allowed separate, detailed agreements. Experience gained in negotiating the contract and operating another institution laid the groundwork for more contract management arrangements.

In August of 1977, Wesley Manor, a 320-unit residential retirement home with 80 nursing facility beds, signed a management agreement with Methodist Hospital. Again, Methodist provided an administrator and service contract for additional management support.

By October of 1977, Methodist Hospital had added a third contract institution. This contract relationship with an 84-bed county hospital showed the most potential for providing good mutual benefits. The county hospital had a viable medical staff which already fostered a physician referral relationship between the two medical staffs which could be expanded and strengthened. Also, the small hospital was constructing a new, complete replacement building.

Methodist Hospital's purpose in undertaking management of other institutions is to develop referral patterns from other hospital medical staffs to Methodist's medical staff. Development of this referral relationship, of course, does not result directly from the management contract or relationship. Rather, as continued medical education programs are developed involving Methodist and the contracted institutions, barriers to referrals are identified and eliminated, and this concerted effort allows physicians from other institutions to become involved at Methodist.

Beyond the direct sharing between Methodist Hospital and contract institutions, Methodist's marketing involves using participating institutions to help develop shared services with other health care facilities. For example, one Methodist hospital program, just being developed, entails the provision of nuclear medicine services to other hospitals through the use of a mobile van. One of the contract hospitals stimulated development of this program because it needed these services and is now helping recruit more small hospitals interested in nuclear medicine. The volume from three or four participating hospitals can be used to justify capital expenditures involved in the program.

May—September 1978: Marketing Research

After 2½ years of marketing its tertiary care services, Methodist Hospital began to assume the private referral center role. The key to this central role is referrals. While Methodist proceeded with its shared services program and management contracts the hospital administration had no specific evidence of the way referral relationships were developed. Hence, Methodist decided to conduct marketing research by surveying referring physicians.

Aimed at physicians in the 34-county area comprising central Indiana, the survey's purpose was to determine doctors' referral patterns, why or how those patterns developed and what problems—both general and specific to Methodist Hospital—doctors encountered when referring patients.

Two sampling approaches were used. First, physicians were selected at random from the entire physician population in this area. However, serious doubts about the expected return rate from a direct mail survey necessitated using a second strategy. The survey instrument was sent to hospital administrators in the area, who asked physicians to complete the surveys at their next medical staff meeting.

Ironically, the first sampling approach yielded a 52 percent return, while the second only netted a 16 percent return. The final total of 185 completed responses were enough to yield statistically valid information.

Survey results were far more informative than original expectations. For example, Methodist learned that in spite of a 700-bed hospital on the east side of Indianapolis and a 600-bed hospital on the northside only one real competitor, the Indiana University Medical Center, challenged Methodist Hospital for any significant amount of referrals. Before the survey, Methodist assumed that these two other large hospitals were significant competitors for referrals from counties two or three removed to the east and north.

Also, the survey showed that Methodist's strength in the referral market, while second to Indiana University Hospitals in the overall 34-county area, was significantly stronger in the first area outside Marion County, the seven contiguous counties, and in the second area, those counties once removed. However, Methodist was second to Indiana University Hospitals in the third area, those counties two or more removed. The difference between Methodist Hospital and Indiana University Hospital in the third outside area was great enough to put Indiana University Hospital ahead overall in non-Marion County central Indiana referrals. The survey clearly showed Methodist which geographic markets were strong, where serious competition existed, and identified the major challenger.

To some extent, the survey explained the geographic differences in Methodist and Indiana University Hospitals' referral markets. It showed that doctors refer patients to Methodist because of specific medical staff members, while they refer patients to Indiana University Hospitals because of its medical center reputation. Clearly, this distinction indicated that Methodist's best short term marketing approach would entail making specific medical staff members visible, and that the hospital's reputation and image as the private referral center had to be solidified on a long term basis.

Methodist also learned that physicians refer patients to other physicians after hearing them speak at professional meetings, lectures and seminars, by past association during their residency, and by personal acquaintance. All other ways of developing referrals, such as "word of mouth" reputation, were much less significant. Obviously, this suggests that encouraging medical staff members to present clinical programming is a good marketing strategy and one which the hospital definitely needs to foster.

While not much has been mentioned about physician recruitment as part of Methodist Hospital's marketing program, it is a very key element and its importance was indicated in the referral survey. Clearly, for a hospital developing its tertiary care role, having the right subspecialist on the medical staff is a must, long before questions of strengthening the doctor's referral network can be dealt with.

Beyond these examples, the marketing research identified Methodist Hospital's strengths and weaknesses which both helped and hindered the referral process. Although undertaken fairly late in Methodist's development of marketing efforts, this research significantly contributed to increasing sophistication of the program and convinced the hospital administration of the value of specific market research.

Methodist is currently conducting a public opinion survey of Indianapolis area residents to identify and evaluate Methodist's community image and determine how that image compares to public opinion of other local hospitals.

January 1979: Results—Programs and Patients

What has been the impact of marketing activities at Methodist Hospital? New revenue programs have been developed. Clinical shared services have been implemented. Methodist has undergone significant market changes in terms of the population served, while it has maintained its traditionally high occupancy rate and stabilized its financial position.

Nineteen shared services arrangements are in affect, including such diverse programs as providing respiratory therapy, remote cardiac monitoring, joint purchasing, and management consulting for outlying hospitals. Three institutions are also under management contracts.

Between 1974 and 1978, the average inpatient occupancy of Methodist Hospital increased 2.3 percent from 84.6 percent to 86.9 percent. As well, the hospital's market has changed significantly. The percentage of patients from Marion County dropped six percent, from 72 percent to 66 percent, while the percentage of out-of-county patients rose from 28 percent to 34 percent. The decrease in Marion County patients is not due to a population loss, but to a population shift and increased utilization of other Marion County hospitals. The increase in out-of-county referrals was attributed to Methodist's more sophisticated services, which reflects the hospital's trend away from primary and secondary hospital services towards secondary and tertiary ones.

Methodist's outpatient volume has increased since 1974, and again, the market from which the patients have been drawn has changed. Referred outpatient visits for sophisticated laboratory and radiology procedures such as brain scans increased six percent, a significant rise. In 1978, 12 percent of all emergency patients came from outside Marion County. Also, 19 percent of the hospital's admissions originated at the emergency department. This compares to the national norm of about 14 percent.

As an inner city institution, Methodist Hospital has aggressively tried to market its tertiary care services, and has successfully maintained its patient volume and financial viability despite a population move away from the immediate vicinity and the growth of newer hospitals. The key effort has been developing more specialized services and seeking broader markets from which to draw patients. These efforts, consciously undertaken to sell Methodist's growing tertiary care role to new markets, emerged over the four-year period from the crisis year of 1974 to 1978.

INDEX

About the Author

PHILIP D. COOPER, Ph.D., is currently Director of Marketing for the O'Connor Hospital in San Jose, California. Prior to faculty and teaching positions at the University of Virginia, Memphis State University, and Penn State, he served in brand management for Hershey Foods Corporation, sales promotion for Pillsbury, and sales for Procter and Gamble.

Dr. Cooper has focused on the use of marketing in a health care setting since 1971. He has written extensively in the area. One article, "Marketing: Entry Points and Pitfalls," which was coauthored with Richard Maxwell, was one of the six selected by the American College of Hospital Administrators for the Hayhow Award and appeared in the 1979 volume of *Hospital and Health Services Administration*. He also has numerous articles in marketing and other business oriented publications.

Dr. Cooper is an active consultant for hospitals, HMOs, primary care centers, and hospital corporations. He has participated in numerous seminars and workshops and has appeared as a guest speaker on the topic of health care marketing and planning throughout the country.